I0766712

CLUB FOOT
Simplified

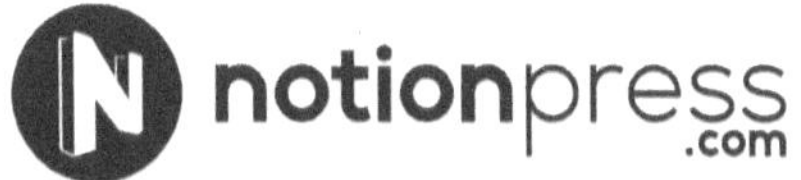

CLUB FOOT
Simplified

DISPELLING MYTHS AND MISUNDERSTANDING
AROUND CLUBFOOT AND ITS TREATMENT

SANTHOSH GEORGE

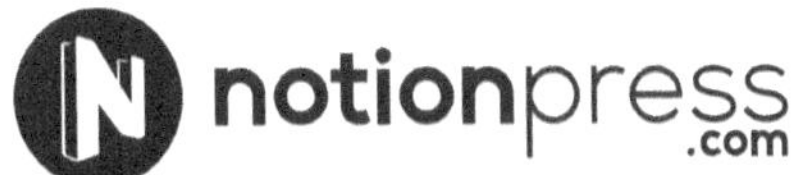

Notion Press

Old No. 38, New No. 6
McNichols Road, Chetpet
Chennai - 600 031

First Published by Notion Press 2016
Copyright © Santhosh George 2016
All Rights Reserved.

ISBN 978-1-946390-07-3

Contents

Contents

Foreword

My involvement with the clubfoot program in India has been one of the most inspiring experiences of my life and career, and at the heart of this is Santhosh George. He has worked tirelessly to create a comprehensive, efficient and effective program to implement 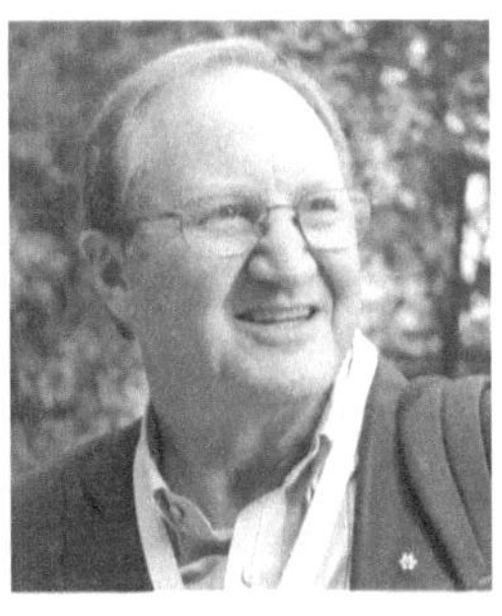 clubfoot training and care in all the states of India in partnership with state governments, hospitals and dedicated professionals, and with the support of several non-governmental oganizations. His passion is to bring compassionate care to every child in India born with the impairment of congenital clubfoot, especially those who are most disadvantaged.

This book tells the story of the development of the clubfoot program in India and explains the care pathway for parents and professionals alike. I know that it is his desire that the awareness of this condition permeates all Indian society and that no child in India suffers disability and no parent suffers heartache, as a result of clubfoot deformity.

It has been my privilege to partner with Santhosh and his team as a trainer of medical professionals and I hope that everyone who reads this monograph becomes more knowledgeable, more caring, and more inspired to see children born with clubfoot deformity cured and set on the journey of a full and productive life equivalent to their peers.

Dr Norgrove Penny
Paediatric Orthopaedic Surgeon
University of British Columbia
Victoria, CANADA.

Acknowledgements

Serving children born with clubfoot is a rare lifetime opportunity for which I am thankful to God Almighty. Seven years back for the first time I heard the word 'clubfoot.' I didn't know anything about this birth deformity when Mr Andrew Mayo the Executive Director of CURE Clubfoot Worldwide, first met me in Delhi. We didn't know where and how to start a program that would impact thousands of children in India annually. Starting from 2009 with the first medical training program in Delhi, today we serve children in 27 out of 29 states in India. I am thankful to the CURE family worldwide for this great experience. Thanks to Mr Jim Cohick who led CURE clubfoot program after Mr Andrew and the present Executive Director, Mr Scott Reichenbach for their trust in me. The CURE India board lead by Dr Belinda Bennet and all the members guided me throughout the growth and spread of our program. What I have written down here is a record of what I have learnt in my association with CURE.

Dr Mathew Varghese's leadership in CURE India enabled the program expand further in India. When I first met him 11 years back at the St Stephens hospital, New Delhi where he was the Director, I never thought that I would have the honour to work with him so closely. He is truly a servant leader, a passionate teacher and a selfless doctor who never sleeps. From Monday to Saturday he is busy either in his outpatient department, standing from 8 in the morning till 6 in the evening without tea or lunch break, or on the surgery day, when he goes on from 8 in the morning to the next day early morning even upto two or three. I learnt about clubfoot mostly from him. I heard all his lectures several times.

I am also indebted to a team of senior orthopaedic surgeons in India without whose help clubfoot program wouldn't have reached its present position. Dr Anil Mehtani, Dr Anil Dhal, Dr Shah Alam Khan, Dr Vikas Gupta, Dr Anil Aggarwal, Dr Rajesh Kanujia, Dr Alok Sud, Dr Shoba Arora, Dr Alaric Aroojis, Dr Gopa Kumar, Dr Ajoy Kr Manav, Dr Mohammed Ismail, Dr Rudra Prasad and Dr Pasupati are few among the leadership faculty team who have selflessly laboured to spread the Ponseti Method in India.

Dr Shafeque Pirani, Dr Norgrove Penny, Dr Steve Mannion, Dr Chris Lavy, Mr Michiel Steenbeek and Dr Joseph Theory are some of the international faculty who encouraged me constantly in our endeavour to see India free from the disability of clubfoot. Timely support from the partners like miraclefeet, Wonderwork, CBM International, ICRC, Rotary International and Inner Wheel are significant. It was such a great honour to sign Memorandum of Agreements (MoU) with Health Department officials in 27 states in India and I am indebted to each of the officials, Health Ministers and staff in Health & Family Welfare and Medical Education Departments.

Cooperation from parents of children under treatment and the sincere service of my colleagues at the national and state offices and the brace production team are equally matchless. Thanks to Notion Press team for the publication support, Vineet Samuel for the sketches and Dr Iris Devadason for meticulous proof reading. Finally thanks to my parents Prof J. George and Mrs Florence Inpam George for their prayers, to my sisters Dr Shanti Dickson, Er Shirly Jacob and Mrs Jayanthi Sunny for their wishes and to my wife Atula Jamir and Son Senup Santosh George for their constant support in making this program successful and this book a reality. I dedicate this book to a world without disability from clubfoot.

Introduction

One regular query we receive from many families is whether pregnancy should be terminated because the child expected to be born has clubfoot. Phone calls, emails and personal visits of parents to our office and clinics are a proof of ignorance of this birth deformity among the general public. It takes time to help young parents understand facts about clubfoot and much more time to help them understand the treatment process.

However when parents know the prevalence of clubfoot and the availability of simple non-surgical treatment for clubfoot, they leave deciding to return with their new-born child for treatment for clubfoot. Myths and misunderstanding around clubfoot and its treatment have to be dispelled. The general public should have access to correct information of this birth defect and the consequence of not treating this deformity soon after birth. This book is intended to raise awareness of clubfoot and its treatment and address this gap of non-availability of sufficient information for general public.

Clubfoot can be treated and children born with clubfoot can lead a normal and productive life. Over 220,000 children are born with clubfoot in the developing world every year. To eradicate disability from clubfoot from the face of this earth, the general public should well know about clubfoot as a birth deformity and its short term treatment and long term follow-up. Clubfoot in a family should not bring shock or social stigma. The right information can dispel myths and misunderstanding around clubfoot and ultimately make clubfoot disability a history. This book offers very vital information parents and the caregivers should know to help children get the best treatment available called the Ponseti Method.

It is important that every child born with clubfoot receives the Ponseti method treatment on time with proper follow up. There are many social and financial reasons why children don't reach the right clinic for the right treatment at the right time. Some parents think that their child is born with polio whereas many others think that birth deformities cannot be treated. Some communities believe that the clubfoot is a curse from God and it should not be treated; the belief is that treating the child born with clubfoot is going against the will of God that could invite the wrath of God. People who are economically weak think that treatment for clubfoot is very expensive and never even approach any hospital or doctors for opinion. Some parents who can afford to spend money look for instant remedy and opt for surgery that ultimately leads to lifetime pain and stiffness and in some cases lifetime disability. Different beliefs and experiences are the result of growing misunderstanding, fear and confusion that still prevail among the people about disability in general and clubfoot in particular.

Why this book?

There are also some reasons related to treatment that keep many children away from any treatment for clubfoot and in some children they end up having incomplete treatment. For example, doctors correct the deformed foot successfully with Ponseti method, but the non-availability of the right and affordable foot abduction brace undermine all their sincere efforts. The corrected foot relapses because of this situation of non-availability of the right foot abduction brace. Doctors and their skills and initial correction do not guarantee completion of treatment for clubfoot. Equally or more important is the maintenance of correction for five years and for this the parent's role in the success of treatment for clubfoot cannot be ignored.

Some parents due to lack of money buy one foot abduction brace and don't take regular follow-up seriously. Those parents, who miss bringing their child regularly, return after six months or one year with a relapsed foot and blame the doctor for not correcting the foot well enough to retain the corrected position. It is not the mistake of the doctor for the child to have relapsed feet, but inability of the parent to buy expensive braces and in some cases the non-compliance of the parents that has failed the Ponseti method of clubfoot management. It is also not just the inability or irresponsibility of the parents that has caused relapse, but the right information on the importance of follow-up that was not shared with them enough to be convinced that has led them to such a situation. **Helping parents understand the chances and challenges of relapse is a very important aspect of clubfoot treatment.** There are also situations where parents want to get the best braces for their children but the proper foot abduction brace is not available in the market.

It is my wish that this book provides accurate information about:

a. the prevalence of clubfoot and
b. the availability of non-surgical methods to successfully correct the deformed foot.
c. The spectrum of clubfoot, the importance of Pirani scoring and long term bracing in Ponseti method are explained here with the hope that it will enhance the quality of treatment provided to children born with clubfoot globally. I hope that these facts will encourage parents to actively participate in the treatment journey with confidence and determination.

1. Spreading Ponseti method globally

Dr Ponseti's dedicated leadership in developing a new method of treatment for clubfoot will be remembered at least until the scientific world finds a way to prevent clubfoot in itself. The Ponseti method has saved thousands of children around the world from a lifetime of disability. The method is very specific and simple yet it has not successfully spread across the globe as it was expected. The Ponseti method explains the simple way to correct the foot with weekly serial casting that concludes with a simple procedure called tenotomy. This corrected foot has to be maintained for four to five years to prevent recurrence and relapse.

Many doctors were given good training in the method yet they couldn't succeed in completing the treatment they initiated in children. Many children abruptly stopped the treatment. Many children got very good casting and tenotomy but did not get the proper foot abduction brace to maintain the correction. The casting and tenotomy get over by 4 to 6 weeks but it is important that the corrected foot is maintained in the corrected position for the next 250 weeks using the proper foot abduction brace. The parents should be given the appropriate information on the long term follow up so that they are convinced, begin to care and remain dedicated.

CURE Clubfoot since 2006 has developed a successful program management model to help children successfully complete the Ponseti method. The CURE Clubfoot program was first developed in Kenya as a national program and then spread globally. Parent counselling, parent teaching materials, refresher training for doctors who are already trained, active ownership of local government, standardisation of documentation, ensuring brace availability, long term follow up, reinforcement of protocol, a system to ensure quality and standard training are some areas to which CURE clubfoot has contributed to take the Ponseti method successfully to corners of the world. I had the privilege to initiate, develop and manage CURE Clubfoot program in India (www.clubfootindia.in) for seven years and here I share the knowledge gained from this unique once in a lifetime journey.

2. Who should read this book?

This book is for mothers, fathers, grandparents or anyone who has a child with clubfoot. Even if parents have not heard about clubfoot, this book will give all the required information to care for their children well enough and save them from a lifetime disability. Accurate information on clubfoot and access to the Ponseti method and proper follow-up can help many children born with clubfoot get the foot corrected, prevent lifetime disability and lead a productive life.

Do NOT get shocked when you come across clubfoot. Clubfoot is not a serious problem; it can be treated with a simple technique using a weekly plaster casting called 'The Ponseti Method.'

First and foremost the intention of this book is to reach anyone who has someone in the family with clubfoot. **Read this book and make sure that the child is getting the right treatment at the right time from the right clubfoot clinic by the right person and gets the right follow-up with the proper foot abduction brace on whichever foot needs cure.** Clubfoot and its treatment are simple and I have further tried to simplify it in this book.

i) For parents:

If you are a parent of a child born with clubfoot reading this book, very carefully make sure to go through the Frequently Asked Questions (FAQ) in detail. The size and fame of the hospital you choose doesn't matter in the treatment for clubfoot; **what matters is the availability of a trained doctor, your determination to get the right treatment using the Ponseti method and your resolution to complete the treatment successfully with minimum five years of follow up with the proper foot abduction brace.** You have an opportunity to enable your child to lead a normal and productive life using an inexpensive but very effective method. In fact the Ponseti method is the only method that corrects the clubfoot with a minor scar and less complication. The Ponseti method requires the active participation of parents for a long time. Your determination determines the success of the treatment. Understand the treatment protocol and make sure that the doctor/care givers provide as it is explained in this book.

There are not for profit organisations leading the management of clubfoot disability eradication program across the globe. Below given are some of the organisations I was fortunate to know and work closely.

www.cureclubfoot.org	www.globalclubfootinitiative.org
www.miraclefeet.org	www.cbm.org
www.wonderwork.org	www.rotary.org

ii) For Clubfoot Program Managers and Counsellors:

You could be a program manager, coordinator or a counsellor involved in the clubfoot program coordination, management or parent counselling. For you this book will serve as a guide in enhancing your knowledge in the understanding of clubfoot, its treatment and the mandatory long-term follow-up. Training doctors alone is not enough to make sure that clubfoot as a deformity and lifetime disability is completely eradicated. Doctors who treat children with clubfoot also have to make sure that correct foot abduction brace is available in different sizes for all children to follow up for five years. The Ponseti method may fail if the parents don't comply with the treatment and bring the child at the appropriate appointments to successfully complete the treatment. It is also very important to document the treatment of each child and the activities in each clubfoot clinic. More important is the regular long-term follow-up for five years. Your role as an integral part of the healthcare team is explained in detail and the information given will give insight on the clubfoot program management.

iii) For Volunteers and Donors:

You could be an active member of any voluntary organisation like Rotary club, Inner Wheel or Red Cross involved in the eradication of disability from clubfoot locally and globally. The information shared here will help you enhance the quality of the clubfoot work you are involved in and ultimately work towards global eradication of clubfoot deformity.

You could be any inspired individual who wants to know clubfoot, causes and consequences of untreated clubfoot and the success of the Ponseti method of clubfoot management so that as a responsible citizen, you can actively participate in the global mission to eradicate disability from clubfoot. You could be any individual or corporate donor wanting to know if clubfoot is an area you could wisely and meaningfully invest to transform lives of thousands of children and change this world for good. In fact in our lifetime we can develop a global network to ensure timely treatment for every child in all corners of every country. We need inspired people to join the global movement. This book will guide to take the global eradication of the disability of clubfoot to a successful conclusion.

iv) For Health Professionals and Community Health Workers:

This book is also for community health workers, volunteers and counsellors, who work with family members of the child under treatment. This book carefully explains in detail, in simple language with less technical terms so that anyone who is looking for details of clubfoot and treatment using the Ponseti method gets true and practical information. The detailed process involved in this short-term treatment that has a long-term follow-up schedule is described lucidly.

Intention of this book; Compulsory and Complete treatment for clubfoot

Since clubfoot deformity and the best treatment available at present are not very well known globally, many children are left without any treatment. Unfortunately many children undergo wrong and expensive treatment that worsens the situation and leads to lifetime pain and complications. There are several families who had to sell everything that they had to raise money to treat a child for clubfoot and yet were not able to give a normal foot experience to their child. This book is intended to dispel the common myths and misunderstanding surrounding clubfoot.

- How can clubfoot be treated?
- What is the Ponseti method?
- Why such a long-term follow up?
- Why a special shoe for my child?

Ultimately the intention of this book is that the information shared here enables every child born with clubfoot in the world get compulsory and complete treatment. Compulsory, so that not even one child is left without treatment. **Compulsory denotes quantity; all children born with clubfoot to get treatment**. Complete denotes quality, so that every child enrolled for treatment gets the foot corrected and the brace follow-up is continued for four to five years. **Complete refers to quality treatment where children successfully complete the treatment**. With compulsory and complete treatment we will be able to see this world free from clubfoot disability. Let every child waiting for treatment and children yet to be born with clubfoot know that there is a cure for clubfoot. Let us share the knowledge; let us together make disability from clubfoot a thing of the past!.

3. Stories that prompted me to write this book

There are thousands of success stories of children that I have come across in my eight years of serving children born with clubfoot. I also heard and came across several heart breaking experiences. Ignorance about the prevalence of clubfoot and the availability of the right treatment has proved very costly to many families. Many children lost their opportunity to lead healed and productive lives. When children are do not reach the designated weekly clubfoot clinics, I know it is ignorance that is keeping them in darkness. When children undergo unnecessary surgery for clubfoot I know it is again ignorance of family members who opt for surgery. When children don't get the right Ponseti Method of treatment again it is the ignorance of healthcare professionals that complicates the treatment method. When parents don't appropriately follow up I know it is the non-availability of the correct and affordable foot abduction brace and the education on the importance of follow-up.

For the majority of parents clubfoot in their child comes as a shocking surprise. A child born with any deformity unfortunately brings social stigma and clubfoot brings more anxiety and helplessness because many have not heard about clubfoot nor seen any children with clubfoot. **When children are born with clubfoot, the foot looks different from how it looks in an adult untreated clubfoot.** Parents think that their child will remain disabled and never be able to lead a normal life. More than the child's disabled foot affecting the life of the child, the family, relationships, happiness and hope gets disturbed with this not-so- well- known or unknown disability.

True story - 1

Sonu was born with bilateral clubfoot in a family in a remote village in the state of Maharashtra. Ignorant of the treatment options but desperate to provide treatment to their son, his parents took him to a doctor for treatment for clubfoot. For every surgery this doctor charged a heavy amount from this poor family and the family had to sell either their cow or goat or any valuable asset they had for every procedure. Finally, they had to sell their only house they lived in to pay the last bill and moved to a roadside hut. The cruelty of the doctor is that in the 3.5 years of prolonged treatment with multiple surgeries he corrected only one foot and told the family to get back to him when they have enough money to correct the next foot! The family never had money for treatment for the second foot.

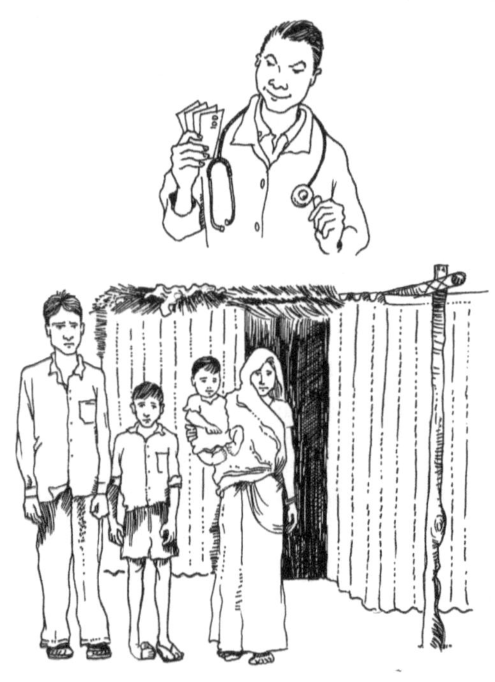

Their second child was also born with bilateral clubfoot. The parents thought that they will never ever try treatment for this child for dearth of money. Fortunately this time a free clubfoot clinic was started by CURE in that town and the parents came across some information in a brochure which said "free treatment for clubfoot," They couldn't believe the CURE counsellor when she said that the treatment is surgery free and is provided free of cost including the special shoes that the child has to wear for five years. Hence proper information can save many lives from lifetime disability and many families from a financial breakdown. The family is happy that Sonu is now ready to walk and run, but the sadness of losing their house for surgical expenses continues to haunt them.

True story - 2

In a remote village in one of the southern states in India, Rena was born with clubfoot deformity. The economically weak family faced severe depression, social stigmatisation and hopelessness. During the first three days this family neither approached any hospital nor did anyone share with them the correct information required. The family didn't know what to do with the disabled child and did not have the courage to face the world's stigma. The father who couldn't face his relatives, neighbours and friends decided to take his life away; he committed suicide. What a terrible story! How could it happen in this age? But sadly it did happen.

The right information about clubfoot and its treatment can save many lives. The mother and child approached a medical college where CURE runs a designated weekly clubfoot clinic. Rena's feet were corrected and she is wearing braces during the night and even during naps to prevent recurrence. Moved with compassion, the CURE counsellor requested the doctor to help this young widow as a result of which the hospital authority gave her a job in the orthopaedic department.

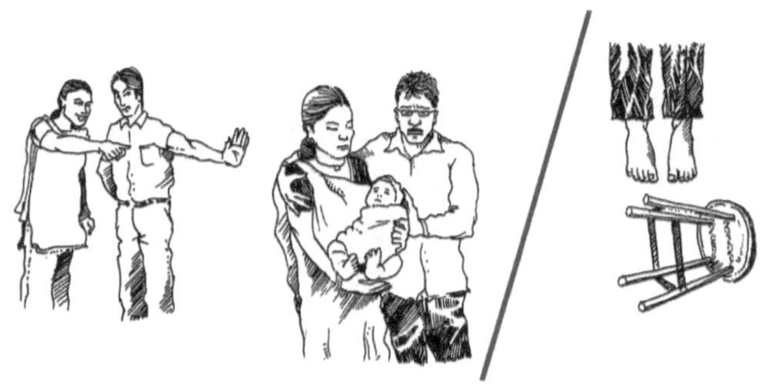

True story - 3

In the capital city of India, Mohini was emotionally devastated when she came to know that the child she had just delivered had some serious birth deformity that was clearly visible. To her misery was added hopelessness from healthcare professionals, to relatives, to friends saying that the child will never be able to walk or lead a normal life. Out of desperation the family members consulted a seer and the seer asked the father Mahesh not to look at the face of his child born with clubfoot for a month! The belief was that if Mahesh looked at the face of the child, the child might die. This father who was a professional photographer couldn't take a single photo of his son for a month. However today the child's feet are corrected and he is a very active child who brings lots of joy to his parents. Myths and misunderstanding regarding clubfoot bring fear and anxiety to many families and communities.

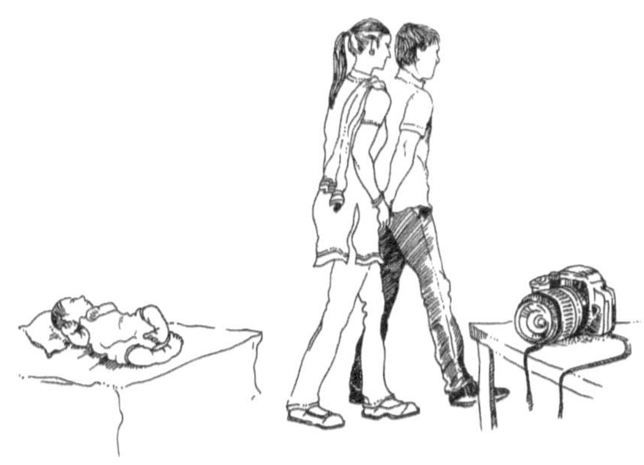

The Uganda Story

I happened to watch a video produced by the Uganda Sustainable Clubfoot Care Project (USCCP). The video depicts some social practices from rural Uganda. It is accepted that any child born with clubfoot should be drowned in any river. When a child is born with clubfoot, the community organises a gathering where the mother and some senior women enact a real tragedy. The Mother will take her clubfoot affected child hung on her back with a cloth to a river and pretend as if the cloth is untied accidently and the child is slipped away. The entire women group will go on an intentionally failed search mission in the water. After this drama for a few minutes they all come out mourning and the entire event concludes with a community dance of celebration of liberation from evil.

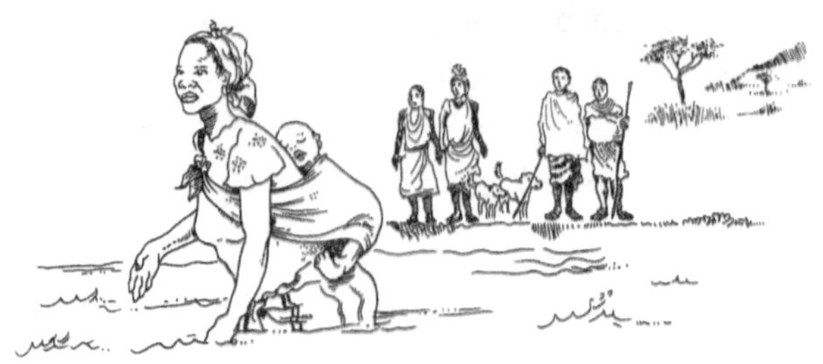

I was told by some mothers in India, who brought their children to clinic for treatment that in many villages in India to a girl child born with clubfoot is thrown in the river. They say that the belief among rural communities is that some evil came through the child in the form of disability and when the child is thrown in the river the evil will return to the river goddess. Few mothers in a clubfoot clinic once said, 'how many girl children could have been saved if only people knew that clubfoot can be treated.' Clubfoot also remains one justification for female foeticide.

Failed treatment story from Ireland and England

A 24 year old girl finally had legs amputated because of unbearable pain as a result of multiple failed clubfoot corrective surgeries. She is originally from Texas, USA and had all her surgical treatment attempts in Ireland suffering 24 years of pain and finally losing her legs. The scientific growth in the field of clubfoot treatment has not reached all children even in the so-called 'developed countries' with more economic progress. If this kind of experience is faced by children born with clubfoot in the so called developed countries, imagine the plight of children born with clubfoot in developing countries with less economic progress. Hope the situation in these countries has changed and presently children are given compulsory and complete Ponseti method of treatment.

A 19 year old girl who had migrated to England from another continent recently contacted me through email. She has clubfeet and some problems related to her hip. She has had 20 surgeries and the pain is still haunting her and she was asking if something could be done in India to get her foot set right that can save her from disability and pain. The Lack of right information and correct treatment can spoil the lives of children, destroy education opportunities and the ability to lead healthy and active lives.

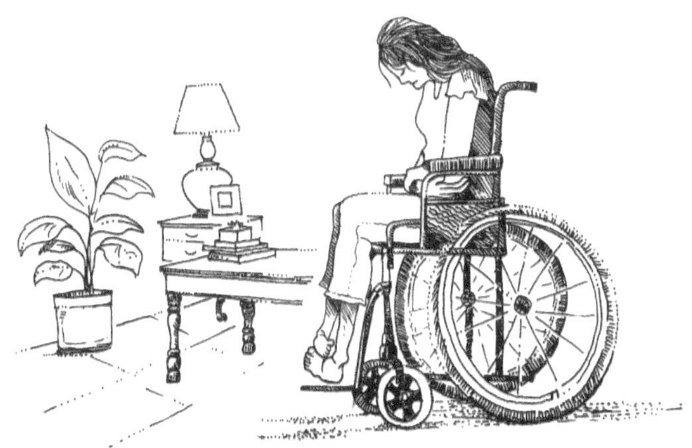

4. Why have I written this book?

My experiences working in Clubfoot India have enabled me to write this book. I have been working for over seven years now with parents of children born with clubfoot, doctors treating children born with clubfoot, networking with government officials for partnership, Rotarians and program managers and counsellors helping children and their parents who successfully complete the treatment protocol for clubfoot. I have personally organised and thus attended 55 medical training workshops on the Ponseti method of clubfoot management and heard the standard lectures so many times. Over 3000 doctors have been trained in these refresher training program in the last seven years. Over 220 designated weekly clubfoot clinics were established in public hospitals and government medical colleges. Nearly 30,000 children have been enrolled for free treatment using the Ponseti method of clubfoot management. Hence, I thought I should share all my knowledge on clubfoot and its treatment in very simple language so that someone somewhere can understand, follow, use and benefit from it.

I have personally led training for the program managers, coordinators and counsellors. It was a privilege to develop and introduce program training materials for clubfoot treatment management and follow up work. In this process of creating training materials, I tried to simplify teaching and learning of the understanding of clubfoot, its treatment and long-term follow-up. I am only sharing what I have learned and experienced in my endeavour to develop a national clubfoot program in India. In this national program at present every month nearly a thousand new children are enrolled for free treatment using the Ponseti method.

I thought, I should write down all I know about clubfoot so that somewhere if a child is given the right treatment and saved from lifetime disability, the purpose of this book is fulfilled.

I. Understanding Clubfoot

5. What is clubfoot? How to confirm a clubfoot?

When a child is born with the foot twisted inward and upward it is clubfoot. Since the foot looks like a golf club, it is called 'clubfoot.' **Clubfoot is always present at birth**. It never occurs after birth. Some children have clubfoot deformity in one foot (unilateral) and the other foot is normal and others have clubfoot in both their feet (bilateral). The ratio between unilateral and bilateral foot is 50:50. Globally clubfoot among boys is more compared to the number of girls born with clubfoot. The ratio is around 60:40 among boys and girls respectively. It is estimated that over 2,20,000 children are born with clubfoot in the in the world every year. The number of children born with clubfoot in each country by and large depends on the population and the birth rate. One or two children per thousand live births are born with clubfoot. However, there could be other specific reasons for higher numbers of children born with clubfoot in different countries.

The technical term for clubfoot is Congenital Talipes Equino Varus (CTEV). Talipes refers to ankle and foot, equino refers to elevated heel and varus refers to turned inward. Congenital means by birth; and talipes, equino and varus are referred to because they are all found deformed in a clubfoot.

There are four areas that are corrected in the same sequence as the acronym 'CAVE.' Cavus, Adductus, Varus and Equinus. Cavus is corrected first by supinating the foot and Adductus is corrected by abducting the foot and in this process of correcting Cavus and Adductus, Varus position of calcaneus is automatically corrected to valgus and finally Equines is corrected with tenotomy. I have explained the treatment process in detail in the Ponseti method session. (page - 32)

The cause for clubfoot is unknown. So, no one can blame either mother or father or anyone else in the family for the child to have been born with this deformity. Among parents who have clubfoot the chances of getting a child born with clubfoot is only 15%. There are many theories on the reasons for clubfoot but till now no theory is proved to be the one and only reason for the cause of clubfoot.

The treated foot is maintained using foot abduction brace for four to five years. If the foot is not maintained in the corrected position, the foot relapses and comes to the original clubfoot position. If the clubfoot is left untreated it leads to lifetime deformity. But if treated with the right method at an early stage (preferably start treatment soon after the birth [but definitely] within the first two to three months) the treatment becomes easy and the child can lead a normal and productive life. The aim is to get the treatment started soon after birth, so that by the time the child is ready to walk the foot is completely corrected and the child has to wear only night and naptime brace.

6. Types of clubfoot

All the clubfeet are not the same. There are four types of clubfoot.

- **Idiopathic Clubfoot:** This is most common type of clubfoot. When clubfoot is the only defect in the child, it is called idiopathic clubfoot. The Ponseti method practiced correctly can correct any idiopathic clubfoot without complication. Idiopathic clubfoot is visible by ultrasound at 16 weeks of pregnancy.

- **Syndromic Clubfoot:** The word 'drome' refers to home. Like aerodrome refers to home to aeroplanes, syndrome refers to home to many symptoms. Syndromic clubfoot refers to several symptoms including clubfoot in a child. So when a child is born with several birth deformities including clubfoot, it is called syndromic clubfoot. Other deformities may include cleft lip, congenital amputation, and rarely cerebral palsy.

- **Neuropathic Clubfoot:** When a child has clubfoot and also neurological defects like spina bifida it is called neuropathic clubfoot.

- **Postural Clubfoot:** This is a very mild clubfoot. The cause of postural clubfoot could be the position of foot in the mother's womb. The proof for postural clubfoot is that the posterior crease will be very visible in such a clubfoot. This type of clubfoot is corrected with a couple of weekly plaster cast. A tenotomy is not required because rigidity of the equines is not present in this type and short term bracing is advised.

7. Clubfoot VS Polio

A majority of the parents mistake clubfoot for polio. They say that the child was born with polio and many of these children in rural places are not administered with polio drops. The risk of these disabled children getting affected with polio is more.

There are five major differences between polio and clubfoot.

   i. Polio affects children after they are born, whereas clubfoot is a birth deformity where children are always born with clubfoot; never after birth.

   ii. Polio is a virus but the cause for clubfoot is still unknown.

   iii. Polio can be prevented since the cause is known, whereas clubfoot cannot be prevented since the reason is still unknown.

   iv. Polio cannot be treated or corrected completely whereas clubfoot can be treated with over 95% success.

   v. Polio may affect the whole leg and upper limbs whereas in clubfoot only the foot gets affected and deformed.

8. Myths and Misunderstanding

i. The most common mistake is saying "The child has to be at least three to four years for any treatment so wait and don't try any treatment at the neo-natal stage," This is totally wrong. In fact children born with clubfoot should start treatment soon after the birth, preferably within the first three months. The point is that the child's deformed foot should be corrected before the child starts walking.

ii. Next, "Surgery is the ultimate treatment for any disability related to bone and not simple 'non-surgical' method, so opt for surgery even if it is expensive," People have this misunderstanding that anything related to disability has to undergo surgery and it has to be expensive, a major surgery which might prove fatal. So out of fear of expense and complications in surgery many parents ignore/neglect clubfoot in their child. **Fact:** The Ponseti Method is globally accepted as Gold Standard for treating children born with clubfoot.

iii. "The more we pay the better treatment we get. So go for more expensive options among the available treatment for clubfoot," **Fact:** The non-surgical Ponseti method is available free of cost in public hospitals whereas in some hospitals treatment for clubfoot is very expensive and comes with assurance of instant correction through surgery. There is a misunderstanding that the more we pay the faster and better is the correction. This is wrong; in fact surgery disrupts joints, spoils the foot and many children suffer pain and stiffness and relapse after very expensive surgery. (refer FAQ session to know why surgery for clubfoot is not good scientifically)

iv. "The disability in the child is caused by something the mother did while she was pregnant. So the mother is the reason for a child with deformity," **Fact:** The reason for clubfoot is unknown till today and so no one should be blamed. Mother cannot be blamed if the child has clubfoot. Some belief is that the mother would have done something that she is not supposed to be doing on a new moon day etc.

v. In India one reason to put all the blame on mothers is to ensure that the parents of the mother pay for all treatment related expenses. When the time come for delivery it is customary that the wife goes to her mother's home. The expenses involved in hospitalisation for delivery is referred to as the burden of 'second dowry.' When a child is born with clubfoot, the mother's parents have to find money for the third dowry, the expenses involved in the treatment for clubfoot. In many occasions the husband's family insists that their grandchild has expensive quick remedy.

vi. "Clubfoot being a congenital deformity (by birth) should not be treated, because God has given this situation in life if altered, we are inviting divine anger," **Fact:** This is common in rural areas but awareness on inexpensive and successful treatment is changing this misunderstanding among several communities. People have started thanking God for the best treatment received by their children.

vii. "After plaster casting, treatment is complete and no need to wear special shoes (foot abduction braces) because the foot now looks normal," **Fact**: It is important that the corrected foot has to be retained in foot abduction brace.

viii. "If there is any relapse after a successful Ponseti method correction, the only way to correct the foot is through surgery," **Fact**: Ponseti method can very well correct a relapsed foot. In fact to correct a relapsed foot is easy and, only requires a couple of casts to bring the foot back to a normal position. It is very important that the relapse is identified and treated on time.

ix. "Any brace available locally is good enough for maintaining correction," Many parents are asked to buy a Dennis Brown splint for their child with clubfoot. The function of Dennis Brown splint is different from foot abduction braces available for clubfoot. The Dennis Brown splint has external rotation of 15 degrees whereas in the correction of clubfoot the foot has to be kept in 70 degree external rotation (abducted position). **Fact**: A specially designed brace like Steenbeek foot abduction brace or other similar specially designed brace with 70 external rotation must be used to maintain the correction achieved by the Ponseti method.

x. "The child has been born with polio so there is no treatment available. It is impossible to correct this deformity," Parents misunderstand clubfoot for polio. **Fact:** Polio is a virus that affects children after birth whereas clubfoot is a birth deformity that cannot be prevented but can be completely treated.

xi. "Girl children with clubfoot deformity should be terminated or aborted," The misunderstanding is that if she is allowed to be born she will be a burden for the family. In the Indian context girl children are considered a burden because of dowry and with disability in a girl child people decide to better terminate the female foeticide than allowing her to suffer. So termination of pregnancy for a female foetus with clubfoot is justified. **Fact:** Every child has the right to be born and get the right method of treatment.

xii. "Let the clubfoot deformity remain at least partially so that the child will get a job in the reserved category of person living with deformity," Intentionally permitting the disability to remain in children is not at all good and advisable. **Fact:** Justice to the child is to get the foot completely corrected and made normal at an early age. It's the right of every child to get the foot corrected completely.

II. Treatment for clubfoot

9. Ponseti Method; The Gold standard treatment method for clubfoot

The Ponseti method is the only method available presently to correct the foot in such a way that the foot is flexible, scar-less, painless and normal in appearance and use. The Ponseti method is named after a Spanish orthopaedic surgeon Dr Ignacio Ponseti who developed and practiced this conservative method while serving children at the University of Iowa in the USA. Surgical correction used to be a very popular method to treat clubfoot. A non-surgical method developed by Dr Kite became popular in 1920s and 1930s. Dr Ponseti's further research on the kinematics of the foot helped him modify Dr Kite's method by suggesting, (i) the head of the talus bone as the fulcrum (Kites method used calcaneus as fulcrum). (ii) Dr Ponseti also advocated the importance of tenotomy for all children (except postural clubfoot) and (iii) further reinforced the use of a long term foot abduction brace to prevent recurrence.

The advantage of the Ponseti method is that the child's foot is corrected within four to six weeks, remains normal looking, flexible, pliable and if the foot is maintained well without any recurrence for the first five years, unnecessary complications could be prevented for a lifetime. Often the child's foot is so well corrected with this method that these children can play, run, walk, dance like any other children born without any birth deformities.

The Ponseti method is widely known as a non-surgical method. It is a method where the foot is corrected with regular weekly gentle manipulation and plaster casting for approximately four to six weeks. The final cast is given after a simple procedure called tenotomy (cutting of tendon). Once casting and correction is complete, the child will need to wear special shoes (foot abduction brace) for four to five years to prevent any relapse or recurrence.

Weekly Manipulation and Plaster Casting:

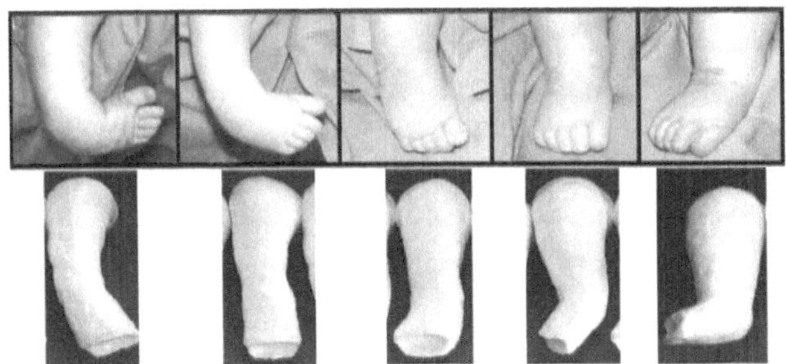

Manipulation and Casting

Gentle manipulation to bring the affected foot to a normal position is the beginning of the Ponseti treatment. The correction is achieved gradually through weekly manipulation and plaster casting. For both the manipulation and plaster cast, the fulcrum remains head of talus bone. Each week after a few minutes of gentle manipulation, a plaster cast is carefully applied to keep the foot in the manipulatively achieved corrected position. There is a very specific hand position that has to be followed while manipulating the foot. Healthcare professionals who attend formal training on the Ponseti method are taught the details of hand position, gentle manipulation and firm (but not so tight) casting from toes to groin. While manipulation and casting, the right foot is held with the left hand with thumb on head of talus. Left foot is held with the right hand with the thumb on the head of talus bone.

After a week, the foot under treatment is again gently manipulated again with head of talus bone as the fulcrum. The foot continues to be gently manipulated to gradually bring it to the normal position. Every week for the next four to six weeks the foot is manipulated and a full leg cast applied. The manipulation is very gentle and the cast is given very carefully from toes to groin so as to successfully get complete correction at the end of casting phase. Generally this weekly cast phase takes four to six weeks. The number of casts may increase or decrease based on the spectrum/type of clubfoot and the age of the child at the beginning of the treatment.

Cast removal and New Cast Application

After every cast, the following week on the same day, the cast is carefully removed by soaking the plaster in warm water. Parents are taught the art of unrolling the plaster by the counsellors. To easily unroll the casting the ends of plaster rolls are gathered and kept in such a way that the parents can identify them and remove them without any efforts. The time between the removal of the old cast and application of the new cast should not be more than 1 or 2 hours. So it is important that the new cast is applied soon after removing the old cast.

The Ponseti Treatment Process and Procedure

Let me explain the Ponseti manipulation and casting in detail. The purpose of the manipulation and casting is to correct the first three aspects of clubfoot as described by the acronym CAVE. (Cavus, Adductus, Varus and Equines). The correction is carried out in the same sequence as in the acronym CAVE. Cavus, Adductus and Varus are corrected first with manipulation and casting. Equines is corrected with a tenotomy. Treatment intends to correct these four deformities gradually and sequentially. Let me explain each one of these deformities in a clubfoot.

    a. **Cavus:** In clubfoot the forefoot is bent downward creating a shape of a cave. The foot looks like a cave. This deformity is corrected first by supination, with the talar head as the fulcrum the great toe (first ray) is raised with middle finger. So after applying the first plaster cast, the clubfoot foot may appear worse than how it looked before the cast. This manipulation is done intentionally to correct the cavus.

b. **Adductus**: In a clubfoot the foot is bent inward. The front of the foot (forefoot) turns inward bringing all the toes closer to the sole and heal. 'Adduction' is bending inward and the opposite term 'abduction' is bending outward or external rotation. Adductus is corrected by manipulating and stretching the foot externally. The middle finger again raises the great toe (first ray) and the pointer finger externally rotates (abducts the foot). Remember the fulcrum remains the head of talus.

c. **Varus:** The bone we feel in the heel, is called calcaneus. This bone is in a wrong position clubfoot and it is called Varus. So in clubfoot when we touch the heel, we do not feel the bone – the calcaneus. When cavus and adductus are corrected by supination and abduction respectively, the varus comes to valgus position automatically. This happens because the movement of one bone affects the position of other bones in the foot and this natural mechanism is called kinematic coupling. Varus is not corrected by any effort in Ponseti method but is automatically corrected as the other bones come into alignment.

d. **Equines**: In clubfoot the tendon in the back of the foot is short (very visible in unilateral clubfoot) and if not treated the weight of walking goes to the toes. This is called Equines and is corrected by a procedure called tenotomy. Tenotomy is the cutting of the tendon. The tendon is cut with local anaesthesia and the cut is so small a stitch is not required. The tendon that is cut regenerates naturally in 3 weeks. In postural clubfoot the equines requires no correction so a tenotomy is not given to those children with postural clubfoot.

Commandments while practicing Ponseti method[1]

These are strict instructions to the doctors and other healthcare professionals involved in the treatment of clubfoot especially to those who apply plaster casting to correct clubfoot. If any of the commandments are ignored the Ponseti practitioners are committing, 'common mistakes in Ponseti method of treatment for children born with clubfoot.'

i. **Thou shall assess and score** every child during every visit using the Pirani Score.

ii. **Thou shall perform tenotomy** in 90 - 95% of children.

iii. **Thou shall be gentle in correction** and maintain the average number of casts to less than eight.

iv. **"Thou shall not pronate"** but only supinate so that the cavus is corrected before correcting adductus.

v. **Thou shall not touch the calcaneus** (fulcrum to be talar head always) and varus gets corrected automatically with the correction of cavus by supination and adductus by abduction.

---

1 Dr Mathew always reminds these points in medical training and I have only reproduced here.

vi. **Thou shall not correct equines by manipulation and casting**. Equines has to be corrected only by tenotomy. If equines is corrected by forceful manipulation and casting, the foot will go to rocker bottom shape.

vii. **Thou shall not ignore the child after casting and tenotomy**. Parents should be guided to follow up for five years of bracing to prevent relapse.

10. Phases & Stages in the Protocol for Ponseti Method of clubfoot treatment

There are two phases in Ponseti method. **The first phase is called the corrective phase** and the **second phase is called maintenance phase**. In the first phase, there are two stages. The first stage begins with weekly manipulation and plaster casting and the second stage includes the tenotomy and the three weekly cast.

Look at the diagram, during the corrective phase children are given weekly casting for four to six weeks. Week after week new plaster cast is applied and the number of casts could decrease or increase based on the spectrum of clubfoot and the age of the child. When the midfoot score is less than or equal to 0.5 and the hind foot score is less than or equal to one the foot is ready for tenotomy. The cast after tenotomy remains for three weeks. This concludes the second stage in the first phase. So in the first phase, the treatment includes weekly gentle manipulation, plaster casting and tenotomy.

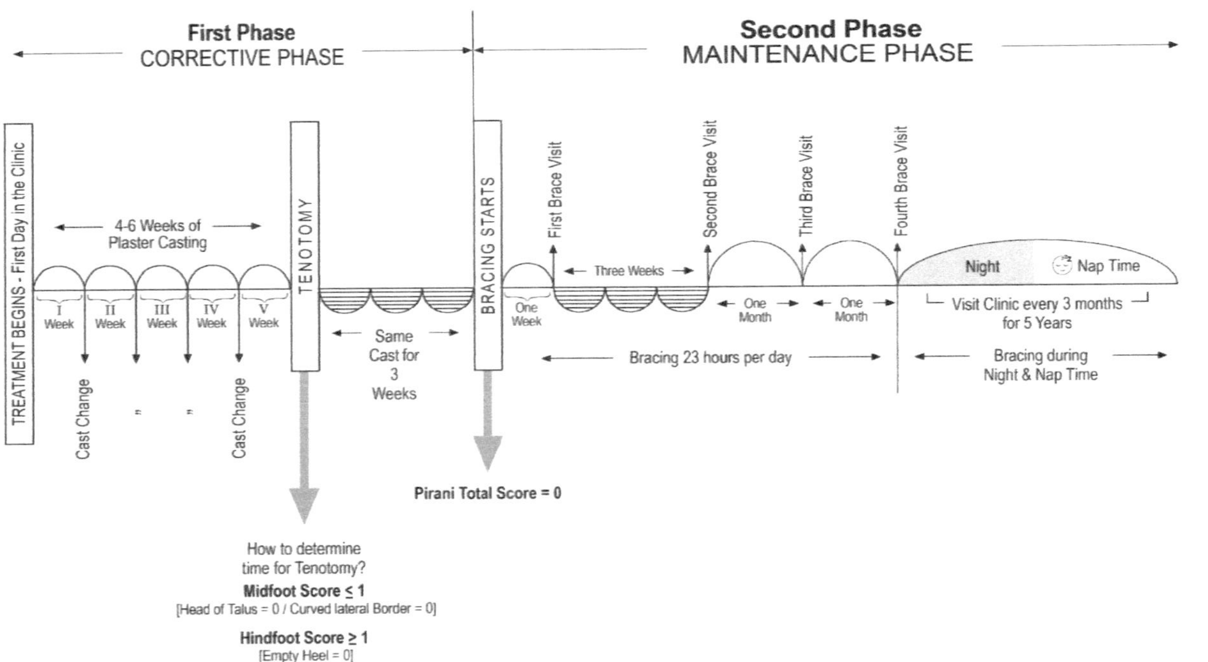

First Phase
CORRECTIVE PHASE
Second Phase
MAINTENANCE PHASE
TREATMENT BEGINS - First Day in the Clinic
4-6 Weeks of Plaster Casting
I Week
II Week
III Week
IV Week
V Week
Cast Change
"
"
Cast Change
TENOTOMY
Same Cast for 3 Weeks
BRACING STARTS
Pirani Total Score = 0
How to determine time for Tenotomy?
Midfoot Score ≤ 1
[Head of Talus = 0 / Curved lateral Border = 0]
Hindfoot Score ≥ 1
[Empty Heel = 0]
One Week
First Brace Visit
Three Weeks
Second Brace Visit
One Month
Third Brace Visit
One Month
Fourth Brace Visit
Bracing 23 hours per day
Night
Nap Time
Visit Clinic every 3 months for 5 Years
Bracing during Night & Nap Time

The second phase is called maintenance phase. In this phase, the foot that is corrected with manipulation and casting is maintained using foot abduction brace. This bracing phase or maintenance phase has two stages. The first three months constitute the first stage, where the child has to wear the brace for 23 to 24 hours a day. The brace is removed only if it is required during feeding, bathing or changing. The duration of time the child is left without bracing should not be more than an hour.

In the second stage of the maintenance phase, the child has to wear the brace for night and naptime. Why night time bracing? Because it is at night when the human bone grows we want to make sure the bone grows in the corrected position. Then why is naptime bracing insisted upon ? When children are given bracing both at night and naptime, the children associate wearing of brace with sleep and there is better adherence by the parents to keep the bracing protocol. When children are given the brace only at night, the child prefers to sleep longer hours during the day (when the foot is left free) and the night sleep gets disrupted. When children are given bracing for the first time, generally first two day and night most of the children cry and resist leaving the foot in the bracing position. To avoid such situation, the child is given the brace both during night and daytime sleep. If the child does not wear the brace according to this protocol, there are definite possibilities for relapse and the corrected foot goes back to the original clubfoot position.

When children are given the brace for the first time they will often resist and cry for first one or two days but then they get used to it. Parents have to be careful to understand the nature of the crying. If the child is crying because of first time brace and annoyance or the child is crying because of some serious problem with the brace? Parents should be careful not to remove brace carelessly when children cry or ask to remove the brace. Once the brace is removed with crying, there are chances that the child will cry every time and the protocol may get disturbed. However if there is any discomfort, bruise or blister the parent should consult the doctor and find a solution to the problem and once corrected continue the brace protocol carefully and strictly to avoid recurrence.

It is important that the parents understand all the four stages (two stages in first phase and the other two stages during the second phase) in the treatment for clubfoot and follow them without any compromise or change. This protocol has been tested for over fifty years and has proven to be very successful in thousands of children who are now adults leading productive and normal lives. Many of the children treated with Ponseti method have grown to become very successful sports persons, athletes, politicians and business leaders.

11. The Pirani Score

Dr Shafique Pirani[2], is a committed orthopaedic surgeon who spends a lot of time learning, researching and teaching about clubfoot worldwide. Pirani score is a common clubfoot assessment language to understand severity of the deformity and the progress of treatment. It

---

2 Dr Shafeeque Pirani's grandparents migrated to Uganda from Gujarat and later the family moved to the UK and at present Dr Pirani lives in Canada.

is like sizing in the clothing industry. There are different sizes in shirts and trousers and general terms like 'I want a big shirt or a small shirt doesn't make any sense for the seller.' But if someone asks for a XL or XXL or Medium shirt or Large, the seller will understand more clearly what the buyer is asking for. Similarly general statements like 'I am treating a severe clubfoot in my clinic,' 'my child's clubfoot is very minor' do not make any sense in the assessment, understanding and treatment of clubfoot.

If a doctor says that, 'I am treating a child who recorded 6 points in the Pirani score initially and has come down to 2.5 in pirani score after three weekly casts,' does make sense. The Pirani scores and points are universally known at least to doctors who are trained and are familiar with clubfoot treatment and programs. The Pirani score helps senior doctors to teach and train the junior colleagues various stages in the treatment for clubfoot. Pirani score help the Ponseti practitioner successfully use the method and conclude the treatment and long term follow-up.

Use of Pirani Score

The Pirani score helps:

1. practitioners understand the severity of the clubfoot deformity.
2. record the progress of the treatment.
3. determine the time for tenotomy. When the hind foot score is more than one (with empty heel is zero) and the midfoot score is less than one (with head of talus and curved lateral border score zero) it is time for tenotomy.

4. understand if it is time for providing foot abduction brace. Foot abduction brace is given only when the total pirani score is zero. That means all the deformities have to be corrected by manipulation, casting and tenotomy, before a child is provided with foot abduction brace. **The foot abduction brace cannot correct the deformity and bring the pirani score to zero.** Brace can only maintain the Pirani score achieved by the Ponseti Method.

5. to identify recurrence at an early stage.

6. parents understand the importance of brace compliance. Once the parents know that their child should score zero throughout the bracing period they are very careful. They have to be taught that if their child scores any point except zero in pirani points during bracing, it will result in recast and/or redo tenotomy. The only way to keep the Pirani score zero is by following the bracing protocol strictly.

The Pirani score points

The Pirani score is a common score/number code to help determine the severity of the clubfoot deformity. It is very important that all Ponseti Providers know and use the Pirani score to correct the clubfoot deformity. A score is given after evaluating six locations of the foot that have to be corrected during the course of treatment using Ponseti method. Three areas to be evaluated are in the midfoot side and three in hind foot (behind/back). For each location the affected posture scores one point.

The less affected position gets 0.5 score point and if the foot is in the normal position the score is zero. If a foot gets 6 points in Pirani score that means the deformity is very severe. The purpose of Ponseti treatment cast is to bring the score to zero. **Only when a foot gets a zero in all six areas, is the foot ready for foot abduction brace**.

1	0.5	0
Very Severe	Partially Corrected	Normal

What are the six locations evaluated for the Pirani score?

In the Midfoot (mid as in middle) three locations/ positions evaluated are

   i.   Medial Crease

  ii.   Head of Talus and

 iii.   Curved Lateral Border

In the Hind foot (Hind as in Behind) three location/ position evaluated are

   i.   Posterior Crease

  ii.   Empty Heal and

 iii.   Rigidity of Equines.

To get the Pirani score you first See, then Feel and finally Measure.

The two things to **see** and score are – Medial crease and Posterior crease

The two things to **feel** and score are – head of talus and empty heal

The two things to **measure** and score are – curved lateral border and rigidity of equines.

Midfoot score

a. Medial Crease: Since clubfoot forms a severe cave like position, it results in one prominent deep crease. When a single deep crease is found the Pirani score is one. With gentle manipulation and casting with the foot in supinated position, this deep crease will gradually lessen. Even after the foot is corrected and ready for tenotomy, there are chances that few creases will still remain. That is the reason in the timing for the determination of tenotomy, it is said that midfoot score could be less than one and need not be zero, because there are chances that the medial crease still scores 0.5 and may not come to zero within those four to five or six weeks. When several fine creases remain, the medial crease score comes to zero.

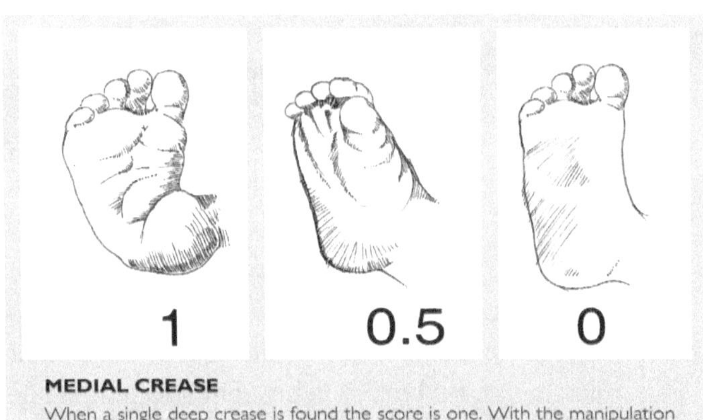

MEDIAL CREASE

When a single deep crease is found the score is one. With the manipulation and casting with the foot in supinated position, this deep crease gradually begin to disappear. Score of 0.5 is when single line is still prominent and may not come to zero within that four to five or six weeks. When several fine creases remain, the medial crease score comes to zero.

b. Head of Talus: In the deformed position the head of the talus is very prominent. For a free kinematic coupling movement, the fulcrum while manipulation and casting has to be the head of talus. And it is important that the head of talus score moves from point one to zero along with the correction of the foot. It is only when the head of talus score is zero a tenotomy can be performed.

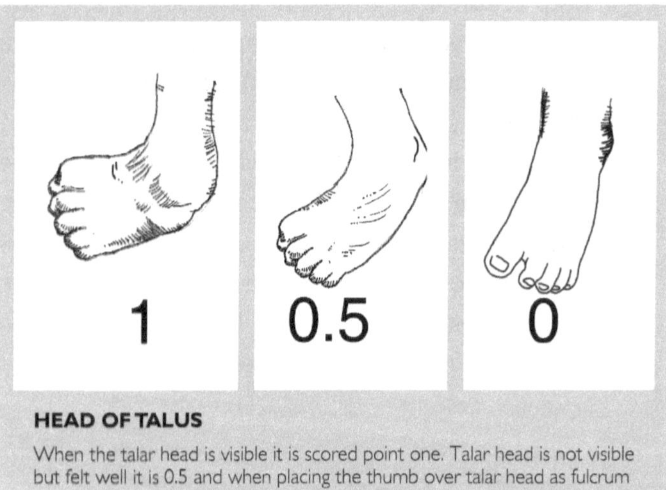

HEAD OF TALUS

When the talar head is visible it is scored point one. Talar head is not visible but felt well it is 0.5 and when placing the thumb over talar head as fulcrum and the talar head has completely disappeared then it is zero.

c. Curved Lateral Border: In clubfoot the midfoot is twisted inward, the lateral border (outside) of the foot is curved inward. In the course of manipulation and casting, when the foot is brought to the normal position it is important that the lateral border is brought straight. While scoring lateral border, it is important that the foot is not held; the foot has to be left free. In the pirani score, when the border is far away from a straight line (scale/pen) the Pirani score is one. If the curved lateral border is coming close to a parallel line, the score is 0.5 and when the lateral border comes exactly parallel to a straight line, the point comes to zero. When the score is zero it means that the foot is now brought to a normal position. It is important to make sure that the curved lateral border score is brought to zero before the tenotomy.

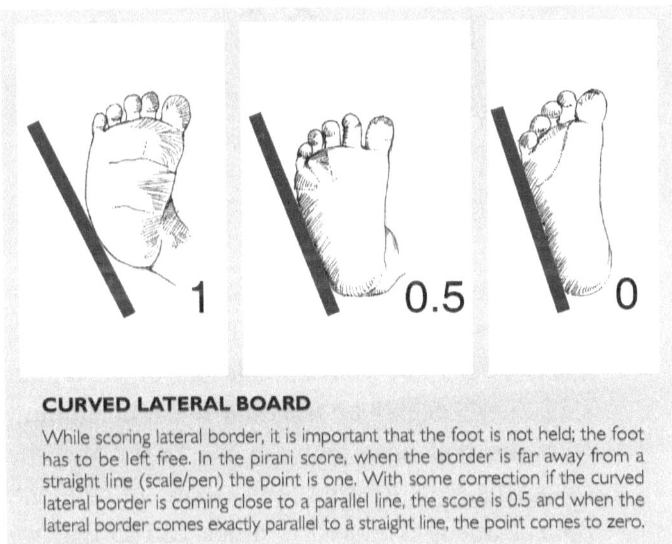

CURVED LATERAL BOARD

While scoring lateral border, it is important that the foot is not held; the foot has to be left free. In the pirani score, when the border is far away from a straight line (scale/pen) the point is one. With some correction if the curved lateral border is coming close to a parallel line, the score is 0.5 and when the lateral border comes exactly parallel to a straight line, the point comes to zero.

Hind foot

a. Posterior Crease: Lines that are seen above heel are called the posterior crease. In clubfoot since the tendon is short, the equines are rigid and instead of several creases, one deep crease appears. The depth of such deep crease is not visible. If there is such a prominent crease the score is a one. If there are two or three not so deep crease, the score is 0.5. no crease is a score of zero.

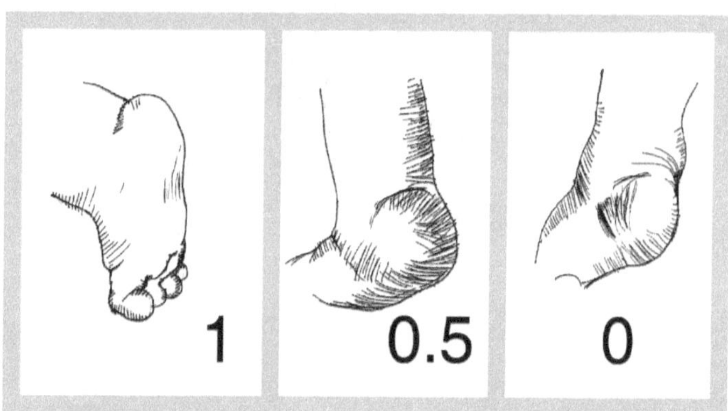

POSTERIOR CREASE

The depth of such deep crease is not visible. If there is such a prominent crease the score point is one. The posterior crease is corrected last, and fine creases appear only after the tenotomy is done. Before tenotomy instead of one deep crease, if there are two or three not so deep crease the score is 0.5.

b. Empty Heel: The score is recorded by feeling the calcaneus (bone in the heel). The calcaneus bone has to be felt not from the sole side or the lateral side, but 45 degree on the hind side. The amount of tissue and flesh between the finger and the calcaneus bone determine the score. In clubfoot, the calcaneus is moved to a position so that we won't be able to feel it well because of the tissue. So when we try to feel the calcaneus, we don't get to feel the bone. It is technically called 'empty heel.' However when the cavus and adductus are corrected, the calcaneus gets corrected automatically and the heel bone begins to be prominent.

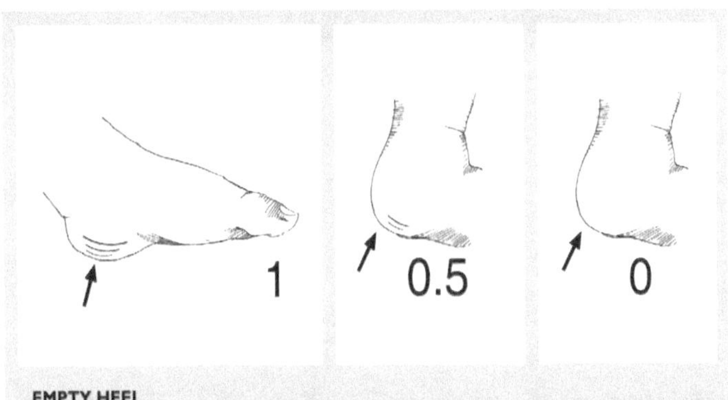

EMPTY HEEL

If the feeling of calcanium is as soft as chin or heel in your palm, the score is 1 and if the feeling is as soft/hard as in the tip of nose the score is 0.5 and when the feeling is like forehead and hard then the score is zero.

c. Rigid Equinus: The ankle is so rigid in clubfoot because of the short tendon. Since the rigidity of the equines is corrected with tenotomy the Pirani score of Rigidity of Equines remains one or 0.5 all through the weekly plaster casting. Only after tenotomy will the score go from one to zero. **It is very important to know that the rigidity of equines should not be corrected with manipulation or casting.** If too much pressure is given to correct equines by manipulation and casting, the foot will result in rocker bottom foot or it even leads to atypical clubfoot. After correcting plantar flex the dorsiflexion is measured.

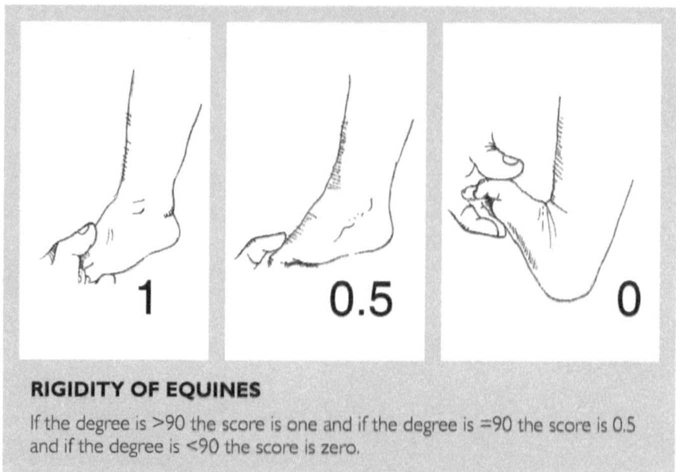

RIGIDITY OF EQUINES

If the degree is >90 the score is one and if the degree is =90 the score is 0.5 and if the degree is <90 the score is zero.

Pirani score during manipulation and casting; points to remember

i. During every visit (Casting, Tenotomy, Bracing and follow up) it is mandatory to carefully evaluate the foot and record the Pirani score

ii. After the first cast (supinated position) the Pirani score may not change and that is acceptable.

iii. However, if there are no changes in the Pirani score during the weekly casting stage for three weeks, i.e. three casts, a senior practitioner should look at the manipulation and cast. No change in Pirani score may indicate bad technique or a complicated foot that require a second opinion. Or there would have been a cast slip that was not noticed. (However among children over two years, there are chances that for the first three to four weeks, the score remains the same and only at the time of the fourth or fifth cast, the Pirani score starts showing different points.

iv. If one foot scores a zero and is ready for tenotomy but the other requires additional casting for tenotomy, both the feet should be casted. The tenotomy should be performed at the same time, so that the feet are prepared uniformly for applying the foot abduction brace.

v. The midfoot score may not come to zero immediately because it takes time for the medial crease to disappear. That is why it is said that the time for tenotomy is when the midfoot score is equal or less than 0.5.

vi. Rigidity of equines is always corrected by tenotomy and not by forceful manipulation and casting. (forceful correction leads to rocker bottom foot)

vii. Varus is automatically corrected to valgus position when the foot is supinated and abducted because of the kinematic coupling structure of the foot.

viii. So, it is important to note that the foot is never pronated and while manipulation or casting the calcaneus is never touched or manipulated.

ix. If the Pirani score is not used, the treatment cannot be considered as the authentic Ponseti method. It is important to score and document the progress of treatment and take informed decisions to move to further phase and stage of treatment based on the pirani score.

x. It should take less than a minute to measure and record the Pirani score. If any doctor or healthcare professional is giving an excuse that time constraints don't allow them to score, please facilitate refresher training so that the Pirani score could be learned and understood and used effectively. The Pirani score is simple and very effective in bringing the Ponseti method to a successful conclusion.

xi. Understanding and use of the Pirani score refers to the confidence level of the healthcare professional in using the Ponseti method successfully.

xii. There are two things you see, two things you feel and two things that you measure to record Pirani score.

12. Tenotomy

Tenotomy is the cutting of the Achiles tendon in the back of the foot to correct rigidity of equines in a clubfoot. The tendon is cut and the foot is flexed and casted to encourage a lengthening of the tendon. The tendon will regenerates natural and lengthen in three weeks, which is why the cast is left on for three weeks following a tenotomy.

The genius Dr Ponseti used his knowledge of the history of prisoners from the Second World War thus when the prisons ran out of space, prisoners were put in locations that had the sea on one side and mountains on the other. The tendons of prisoners were cut by the jail authorities who believed that they would never be able to escape by swimming or climbing the mountain. But they later realised that many prisoners escaped because the tendon regenerated naturally.

For children a tenotomy is a very minor procedure that is easily carried out in the out-patient department or outside the operating room/theatre. Only local anaesthetic is administered and there is no requirement for stitches. Except for postural clubfoot, nearly every child requires a tenotomy. The tenotomy rate in any designated clubfoot clinic should be 90–95%. When tenotomy is not performed, the chances of recurrences are more. Also the Pirani score doesn't come to zero because of the uncorrected rigidity of equines. So without tenotomy the Ponseti method is neither complete nor successful.

How is the time for tenotomy determined?

Equines have to be corrected last after correcting cavus, addatus and varus. The Pirani score is the only and simple way to determine the time for tenotomy. When the midfoot score is less than one and the hind foot score is more than one the foot is ready for tenotomy. Remember to note that the empty heel, talar head and the curved lateral border score should be zero before performing tenotomy. (As mentioned before, in the midfoot the medial crease may remain 0.5 since it takes time to disappear). In the hind foot the posterior crease score may remain 1 and the rigidity of equines is corrected only by tenotomy. So in the hind foot score even when the score is more than 1 the child may undergo tenotomy.

However it is important to note that all the six points come to zero after the tenotomy. If any point remains more than zero, additional casts are applied to bring the foot to zero Pirani score before applying the brace. In some children redoing tenotomy is also possible and done

It is important to note that 70 degree abduction (external rotation) is genuinely required before the child is given foot abduction brace. There is a misunderstanding among Ponseti practitioners that mild deformity could be corrected with foot abduction brace. This is wrong. The pirani score has to be zero before applying a brace. **In other words the foot abduction brace is given to normal foot and not clubfoot.**

III. Follow-up after Ponseti Treatment

13. Foot Abduction Brace

It is worth repeating this statement, foot abduction brace is given to fully corrected foot (normal foot) and not clubfoot (deformed foot). Half corrected or uncorrected foot cannot be corrected with the help of foot abduction brace. Manipulation and weekly plaster casting gets over in an average of four to six weeks; but bracing has to be continued for another at least 250 weeks! In the treatment for clubfoot every step i.e. manipulation, casting, and bracing are all very important and nothing can be ignored or considered insignificant.

Also remember that children do cry for the first two to three days when the brace is worn.

- Allow the child to play with the brace even during the casting period to get familiarised for few days before the child is asked to wear it.
- It is important that the parents do not remove the brace in response to child's fussing or mild crying.
- It is very important to know that the foot abduction brace has to be tied tight ensuring to

avoid friction between the skin and the leather. The brace should not be tied so loosely that the purpose of keeping the foot in corrected position fails nor tie too tight that the foot starts swelling.

- Always remember to have patience while putting the brace. Never give any feeling to the child that it is unnatural that the child has to wear brace.

- Never use the brace to threaten the child; ("If you don't eat food, I will put brace now!) Such statements create negativity among children towards brace.

Choosing the right foot abduction brace and using it as per the protocol is the key to successful conclusion of clubfoot treatment. The doctor could be very good, the casting given the best as possible, tenotomy was done and all went well and the foot was corrected. But if the brace is not used well, the foot will come back to the original clubfoot position. To bring any change again in the foot, the same manipulation and casting treatment has to be initiated including tenotomy. And remember this time the child has grown big and casting could be very uneasy to the older child and difficult for him/her to carryout daily activities. It is always better to treat the child very young and complete the bracing protocol before the child is five years old.

Protocol for bracing is that the child should be given bracing 23 hours a day for the first three months and the next five years the brace has to be worn night and naptime. Remember there is no alternative to bracing but:

- patience from parents,
- close follow up from doctors and counsellors

These are very important during the long term bracing follow up.

14. Access to standard quality foot abduction Brace

Casting corrects the deformed foot and Bracing maintains the corrected foot. Maintaining the achieved correction is the key to success in the Ponseti method. Well reknowned and experienced doctors may provide the best cast, best tenotomy and achieve almost near normal correction but if this corrected foot is not maintained using an appropriate brace, the foot will relapse. Access to the right brace for four to five years after the initial treatment is crucial. **Corrected foot not kept in the corrected position with a brace will relapse and become clubfoot again**. When there is a relapse, the child has to once again start treatment with weekly manipulation and plaster casting. By now the child has grown big and managing a grownup child with cast on both the feet is very difficult compared with a new born baby or any child below one year. So access to good foot abduction brace is the right of the child and very important to successful conclusion of the treatment.

Braces in the market range from Rs 600 to Rs 60,000. However what is important is if the brace has:

a. Seventy degree external rotation.
b. Inspection hole to see if the heel touches the sole well enough.

    c. 15 to 20 degree dorsiflexion so that the degree of heel remains <90.

    d. Light weight (child friendly).

    e. Locally made and easily available and accessible.

Please remember that immediately after the tenotomy cast is removed, the foot has to be in the brace. Just as **the time between the removal of old cast and application of new cast should not be more than one hour, the brace also should be worn without much time gap**.

The trend is that parents with less economical resources manage to buy one pair of foot abduction brace. Since the foot looks normal at this stage of treatment, parents don't understand the importance of repeatedly buying the brace. Parents doubt the persuasion of the brace seller thinking it's for profit that he is forcing them to buy more braces. The less income families have to be supported with free brace to confirm that they ensure compliance.

15. Importance of long term follow-up

Every child who does not get proper bracing ends up with a relapsed foot. Having learnt that long term bracing is important to maintain the correction, it is the duty of responsible parents, sincere doctors and committed program managers to make sure the child is given proper special shoe that keeps the foot in the corrected position.

The treatment process does not stop with the correction of the foot. The foot that is corrected using manipulation and casting has to be maintained at least four to five years. Scientifically it has been proved that once the foot is maintained for five years there is very little or no chances of relapse.

Relapse is directly linked to compliance and cooperation of parents. Dr Ponseti and other senior doctors have over and again researched on the need for foot abduction brace and came to the conclusion that every child born with clubfoot and undergone Ponseti method of treatment requires minimum four to five years of bracing. The foot has to be kept in abducted position with dorsiflexion night and naptime. Neither the doctors, nor the parents or the program managers or counsellors should try to test skipping of bracing in any child. The result of such testing is relapse and the child has to again start the treatment from the beginning; i.e. manipulation, casting, tenotomy and again bracing. There is no short-cut to maintain the correction, so please do not experiment or do any research on innocent children.

Availability and accessibility to braces is as important to maintain the correction as having trained doctors and casting materials for plaster casting. Please remember that the treatment begins with weekly casting and it concludes only after 5 years of bracing. The advantage is that after 3 months of 23 hours of bracing it is only night and naptime bracing. We insist that the child wear the brace both night and naptime, so that it becomes routine activity for parents and children to wear the brace and sleep.

16. Managing Relapse

Relapse is when the corrected normal looking treated foot starts bending back to the clubfoot position. Relapse happens gradually and it is important the doctors identify it at the initial stage and start treating it as soon as possible. The reason for relapse is the non-compliance by the parents. They fail to brace the child and the foot that is left without abduction goes to the original clubfoot position.

Relapse is identified by doctors who carefully record the pirani score during every follow-up visit. It is important that the doctors look at the foot carefully and record each of the six pirani scores to ensure that the score remains zero. In case the score is even 0.5 instead of zero, the area that has relapsed should be immediately addressed. There are chances that the rigidity of equines is coming back or lateral curved border is showing some points in the pirani score.

The way to correct relapse is to start casting until the pirani score goes to zero. If there is relapse in rigidity of equines, the only way to correct is to redo tenotomy. Doctors ask if a tenotomy could be performed again. The answer is yes. The time between the first tenotomy and the second or redo tenotomy should be at least six to eight weeks or more. The point to insert the blade to cut the tendon also should be carefully decided. The redone tenotomy regenerates as well as the first tenotomy.

The point is, if there are any compromises in bracing there will be relapse and if there is relapse, it has to be identified early and the treatment has to begin without any delay. The relapsed foot can be very well corrected by the Ponseti method irrespective of the age of the child. The point is to score every time the child comes to the clinic/hospital for follow-up and if there is a change in pirani score start treatment sooner.

IV. Program Model

17. The CURE Clubfoot Management Model

CURE Clubfoot has developed a program management model to successfully manage the Ponseti method of treatment to a successful conclusion. The CURE Clubfoot management model includes a set of best practices that is followed very intentionally.

In the CURE Clubfoot programme model,

i. Children are treated in designated weekly clubfoot clinics, which have a trained doctor, counsellor, enough stock of different sizes of braces, system to document etc. There is a 36 point check list that is followed to check the minimum required essentials in any ideal clubfoot clinic.

ii. A designated weekly clubfoot clinic is not established in any state or country or province unless the respective government or hospital authority signs an agreement with CURE.

iii. A designated weekly clubfoot clinic will not have children enrolled for treatment until it has a trained doctor/healthcare practitioner and a trained counsellor.

iv. Children and parents are not entertained in the clinic unless there are treatment materials like plaster of Paris, soft ban???, tenotomy requirements, foot abduction braces available.

v. Children do not meet the doctor to start treatment unless the standard medical record file has all details about the child recorded.

vi. Children do not get their weekly plaster casting until the medical practitioner records the pirani score.

vii. Parents do not return home from the clinic until the parents are given detailed counselling and are taught all relevant information from the parent teaching brochure with images of treatment progress and a new appointment date as per the treatment protocol written down in the printed brochure.

viii. If any parent misses their appointment opportunity immediately they are contacted by the counsellor and asked and counselled to continue the treatment without any delay. A new appointment is given over the 'phone and reminder calls are made to ensure the child visits.

ix. Enough foot abduction braces of all sizes are stored in all designated clubfoot clinics so that there is no delay or waiting period for any child for any brace size. The day tenotomy cast is removed the child gets the right size of brace before leaving the clinic.

x. Every clinic has a counselling location, cast removing corner and display of clinic timings and helpline number.

xi. Every state in India has 24X7 clubfoot helpline numbers and a toll-free national clubfoot helpline number where parents can always talk to the counsellors to clarify their doubts, share their challenges or confirm an alternate appointment date with the doctor.

18. Ideal Clubfoot Clinic

In any hospital at the clubfoot clinic if children have to get the right treatment and successful follow-up, there are some essentials:

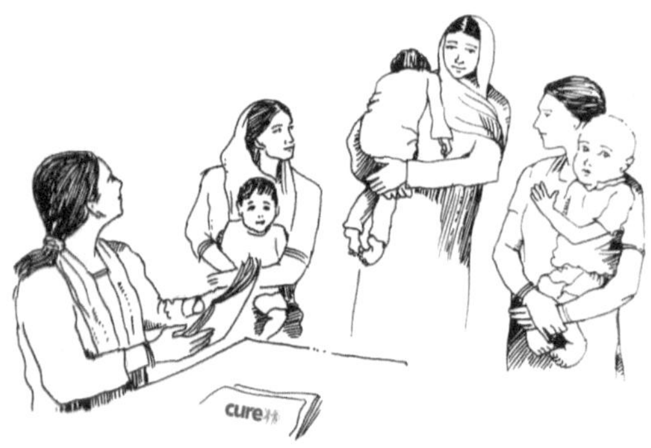

i. Trained doctors who believe and have confidence in the Ponseti method of clubfoot management to be available in the designated clubfoot clinic.

ii. Trained counsellors who know the protocol of the Ponseti method, who have the ability to teach parents on the treatment progress and long-term brace use clarifying their doubts and answering their questions.

iii. Right information to parents on short term weekly plaster casting and long-term bracing is available and a trained counsellor explains them to the parents. (gives out printed materials with images that parents can take away)

iv. Casting facilities that are child friendly with good quality PoP and soft ban.

v. Location to unroll and remove cast with warm water by parents (never use plaster cutter to remove cast; it is noisy, burns the skin and is not child-friendly)

vi. Treatment progress is recorded in detail electronically and also in hard copies to document and use the data for research and quality control.

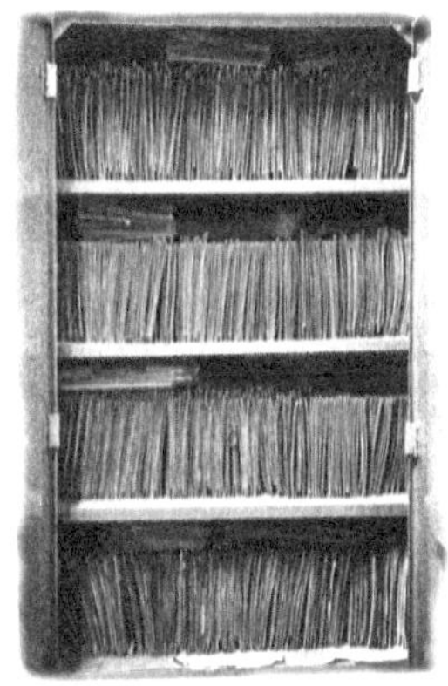

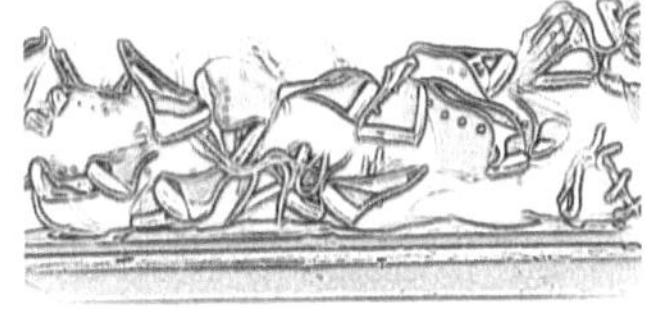

vii. Brace that fits children from 3 months to 13 years to be stored in good numbers, so that children don't wait to get the right brace size.

19. Team work of Doctors, Healthcare professionals, Counsellors and Parents

For a clubfoot to reach a normal foot there are several actions that happen. Every specific step has to be followed, where several professionals get involved in this process that includes weekly manipulation, plaster casting, tenotomy, bracing and long-term follow-up. This long journey is carried out successfully only when we have at least three different groups work as a team. The team includes Doctors and/or healthcare professionals, counsellors and parents.

Three groups of professionals and parents work as a team to provide successful treatment to the child.

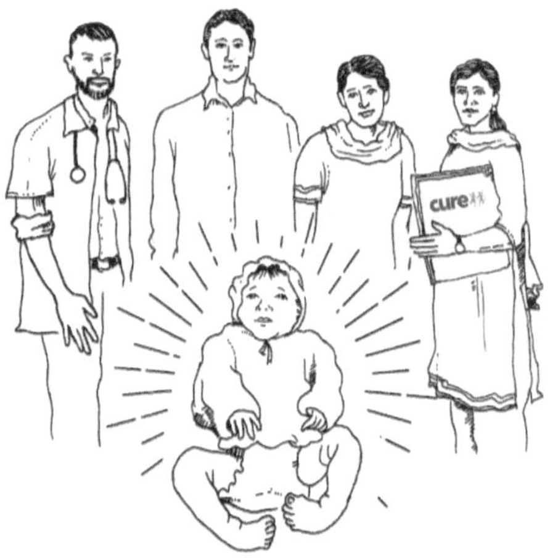

> **Role of Doctors** – Provide gentle manipulation and the best Ponseti cast possible. Perform tenotomy to over 90–95 % of children and record pirani score during every visit. Identify and correct any relapse.

- ➢ **Role of Counsellors** – Ensuring successful completion of treatment in every child by working very closely with parents and the doctors.
- ➢ **Role of Parents** – Determination to treat and correct the foot of the child and comply with the regular and long-term follow-up.

Role of Doctors in an ideal clubfoot clinic

1. Right diagnosis of clubfoot and its spectrum and recording it in the prescribed space in the medical record.
2. Provide gentle manipulation and best casting (from toe to groin) with knee in 90 degree. Neither too thick nor too thin a cast, but enough plaster to hold the foot firm in the corrected position for a week.
3. Record Pirani score during all visits (casting, bracing and follow-up).
4. Perform tenotomy for 90 to 95% of children (except postural clubfoot)
5. Identify relapse and start remedial treatment by providing weekly manipulation & cast and do tenotomy again required.

Role of Counsellors

1. Counselling (active listening) the parents.
2. Teaching parents with the support of information brochure on clubfoot, weekly plaster casting and role of parents in the long-term bracing.
3. Answering questions of parents and clarifying all their doubts

4. Teaching parents the art of unrolling the plaster cast by soaking in water.
5. Call parents if there are defaulters and get them to continue the treatment.
6. Maintain medical record for every child with all information for research and documentation in both hard copy and update in the electronic records.
7. Reporting in the prescribed formats to the doctors, medical director and the line managers.
8. Distribution of foot abduction brace for every child so as to facilitate completion of four to five years of bracing for every child.
9. Raise awareness on the prevalence of clubfoot and the availability of free treatment for clubfoot.
10. Mobilize volunteers, resources and funds to support treatment program.
11. Attend 24X7 clubfoot Helplines
12. Organise parent support group to build a community of parents who support and share experience with each other.
13. Facilitate family therapy sessions for mothers and fathers to share their anxiety, challenges, hope, success and joy.

Role of Parents

1. Believe that the child's foot is going to be corrected with the non-surgical Ponseti method that has 95–98% success rate.
2. Know that the treatment could be started the same week as when the child is born.

3. Have determination and dedication to complete the treatment and follow-up with bracing for at least five years.
4. Care for the cast well so that it doesn't get dirty or break.
5. Learn to unroll the cast by soaking it with warm water.
6. Putting brace to child as per the protocol. First three months 23 hours a day and nap and night time thereafter for four to five years.
7. Care for the brace so that it doesn't get dirty, wet or broken.
8. Know that the correction of the deformed foot is the doctor's duty and maintaining the corrected foot is parent's duty and responsibility.
9. Take the child on time regularly and cooperate with doctors, counsellors and other health professionals in the hospital.
10. Follow the instructions carefully specially on cast care and brace use.
11. Never look for shortcuts and instant remedy to correct the foot that may damage the foot for ever.
12. Share your experience with other parents so that they too follow the treatment protocol and get the benefit of knowledge on Ponseti method.

20. Common errors

Errors occur out of negligence and ignorance. Errors can challenge the quality of correction in the Ponseti method. Errors could occur from Doctor, Counsellor or Parents. Partial understanding of Ponseti method by doctors may not result in good correction; doctors could commit several errors while practicing Ponseti method. Parents and counsellors also could make mistakes that tamper with the success of the Ponseti method. Severe social stigma associated with disabilities and birth defects lead parents to opt for outdated surgical methods. Parents look for instant remedy; they want the foot to be corrected soon so that they can avoid stigmatisation by the society. Negligence of the counsellor may lead to incomplete follow-up of a corrected foot. Errors intentional or unintentional have to be avoided to help children have the best foot that is functional.

Errors by the Doctors/Healthcare professionals

    i.   Providing below knee casts.
   ii.   Casts reapplied once in two weeks or three weeks and not weekly.
  iii.   Changing the priority of correction/ protocol in Ponseti method by sometimes starting with tenotomy and trying to correct equines before correcting other deformities in the clubfoot
  iv.   Casting under general anaesthesia or other sedation.
   v.   Applying more pressure while manipulation that breaks tissues to lead to fibrosis and stiffness.
  vi.   Performing tenotomy under general anaesthesia.
 vii.   Prolonged casting because of unscientific casting or profit motive.
viii.   Providing 20 to 30 weekly cast to one child without a break with no correction achieved yet

not knowing that the number of cast has exceeded several times more than what is required.

ix. Don't know how to identify atypical clubfoot and no experience of treating them.

x. Prescribing 'clubfoot shoes' to wear during day time which do not have any role in the Ponseti method.

xi. Insisting on surgery instead of tenotomy.

xii. Practicing Ponseti method without the knowledge of Pirani score.

xiii. Prescribing foot abduction brace before the complete correction is achieved/before the Pirani score is zero.

xiv. Approving local made brace with no dorsiflexion and no seventy degree external rotation/ abduction.

xv. Not picking up relapses early and not applying cast for relapses.

xvi. Not insisting on follow-up to children for five years.

Common Errors by the Counsellors

i. Not carefully spending enough time with parents on the first meeting. The first meeting of parents with counsellors is very important. Many parents take decision on the kind of treatment they are going to give to their child during such meetings. There are chances that the counsellors can miss the opportunity to carefully counsel the parents on the benefit of non-surgical methods and the success of the Ponseti method. Even after meeting counsellors some parents never return and they choose to go for surgical correction. There are chances that counsellors failed to communicate well enough to help parents understand the right information.

ii. Not following up with the parents who missed the appointment. The counsellor has to immediately find out such parents and get them back to the treatment protocol. Negligence of counsellors can be very costly to the child.

iii. Parents are not taught the right cast care and brace wear.

iv. Not helping parents understand their role during bracing.

v. Not using counsellor's diary to carefully follow-up with the parents.

vi. Not documenting the treatment process.

vii. Not understanding the counsellor's role as 'Ponseti protocol officer' and not helping parents bring children on the appropriate days to complete the treatment.

Common Errors by Parents

i. Not regular in taking child to the clinic thus not following the protocol for treatment. This could delay the treatment process and the best correction may not be achieved.

ii. Carelessness that wets, breaks or dirties cast/ brace of the child: If there is cast break or slip or wet cast, a new cast has to be applied as soon as possible to prevent relapse. Cast break is like leaving the foot without cast. Cast slip could lead to atypical clubfoot. Same importance to be given during bracing phase and the brace has to be maintained clean and dry.

iii. Seeing corrected foot and not continuing long term bracing: With four to six weeks of regular casting, the foot gets corrected. Many parents don't understand the importance of maintaining the correction of the foot by long term bracing and that leads to relapse, where the foot goes to the original clubfoot position.

iv. Seeing other children in the clinic wearing brace, insisting on a brace before completion of casting and correction: Parents see many children in the clinic. Some children just starting the treatment, some in the progress of treatment and others in the final stage of treatment. Parents always want their child in the final stage of treatment that is follow-up using foot abduction brace. Brace is given to children only when the foot is completely corrected; but some parents insist that they get the brace even before the foot is corrected completely with casting.

v. Discontinuing for fear of tenotomy: Parents come regularly to the clinic with their child till the week their child has to undergo tenotomy. Once they hear that the child has to undergo a very minor procedure where the tendon will be cut, parents relate that to surgery and stop coming to the clinic. Such parents who have intentionally stopped the treatment are very difficult to follow-up with and they never return to the clinic. This is an error from parent's side abruptly stopping the treatment.

vi. Insisting on fast remedy for clubfoot fearing social stigma. When a child is born with any birth deformity the parents are blamed. Among parents mothers get more blame and the relatives and neighbours try to find reasons related to the mother for the child to been born with clubfoot. So many parents keep the child in isolation and find ways to get the foot corrected as soon as possible to escape the social stigma. Many children end up having very expensive surgery. Parents don't know the fact that surgery is failure for clubfoot treatment. The common public does not know the fact that surgery is an outdated and failed method to correct clubfoot.

vii. Allowing child to undergo surgical correction for the treatment for clubfoot; There is a misunderstanding prevailing that anything expensive is good compared to anything inexpensive. When parents come across two methods to correct the foot; one very expensive surgical method that promises instant correction and the other very cheap but long term procedure, parents go for the instant and costly. That is an error by parents who have child with clubfoot.

viii. Asking for leaving some uncorrected disability for the benefit of job reservation under disability act: This trend is not very common across the program, but at many locations, parents ask the counsellor to treat the child in such a way that some aspect of the disability remains in boys so that they get a disability certificate that helps them get employed in public sector.

21. Medical training on Ponseti Method of clubfoot management

Since Ponseti technique is a very specific method of manipulation, casting, tenotomy, bracing and follow-up, it is inevitable for any professionals to undergo a recognised training program to understand and master the technique. **The choice of the Faculty members and the content of the training are very important in the success of medical training on Ponseti method of clubfoot management.** Much more important is the hands-on practical sessions provided to the doctors and other healthcare professionals during the training. The practical sessions enhance confidence in the young professionals to successfully employ Ponseti method in the treatment of clubfoot. Theoretical medical training alone doesn't help doctors to be successful in providing Ponseti method to children. Integrating practical workshop on rubber model and children are very important to impart knowledge on clubfoot management to doctors.

Historically it is proved that the trained doctors will be more successful if the children under treatment have access to affordable quality braces. Also the right information to parents on the protocol of treatment and proper follow-up determines the success of the doctor who practices the Ponseti method. It is also important to maintain medical records for every child in detail to understand the progress of treatment. In the training process the doctors are helped to understand the importance of ensuring the right brace to every child they treat and the parents are given the right information and counselling. Doctors who practice Ponseti method should have these additional aspects of the program such as bracing and parent follow-up to be successful in correcting and concluding the treatment to a successful end.

CURE India accepted eleven lectures to be used in all the medical training sessions organised for the doctors from government medical colleges and hospitals. In a training of trainers meet held in 2011, national and International experts representing Global Clubfoot Initiative, CBM International, Ponseti International Association, CURE Clubfoot Worldwide and various senior government doctors who have been practicing Ponseti method participated. Nine standard lectures were accepted by going slide by slide and word by word.

1. Introduction. Clubfoot prevalence - epidemiology
2. Spectrum of Clubfoot (based on symptoms and based on treatment)
3. The Ponseti Method – the Gold method to treat Clubfoot.
4. Kinematics of Clubfoot
5. Pirani Scoring for Clubfoot and assessment
6. Hand Positions for Ponseti Manipulation and Casting
7. Tenotomy

8. Foot Abduction Brace
9. Common Errors in Clubfoot Correction

CURE India has successfully conducted 55 refresher medical training programs where over 3000 orthopaedic surgeons serving in public hospitals and government medical colleges in India participated. These trained doctors have treated over 30,000 children born with clubfoot in the last 7 years.

In addition to the standard nine lectures, two more lectures were added to address specific issues faced by doctors in India. The new topics are

i. Clubfoot in older children
ii. Managing atypical clubfoot, difficult and Syndromic Clubfoot

Attending CURE medical training is mandatory for the doctors who serve children with clubfoot in government recognised centres. This medical training is a one day program with 11 standard lectures and practical s that hands on workshop on rubber models and children. Tenotomy is also demonstrated on children to gain confidence among the new generation doctors.

Doctors through the training are equipped to give

a. Gentle manipulation with head of talus as fulcrum with the right hand position.
b. The best Ponseti cast possible (toe to groin with knee in 90 degree)
c. Pirani score children during all clinic visits,
d. Perform tenotomy to 90 to 95% children (with local anaesthetic),

e. Identify and correct relapse at an early stage.

f. Follow-up children for five years.

Doctors are also given lectures on importance of parent teaching and the role of counsellors in the successful conclusion of the Ponseti method. Every doctor who attends the training gets support of a trained counsellor in the designated clinic. Braces are distributed free of cost to children until completion of five years of follow-up. Further, medical records are maintained for every child electronically and manually in hard files in each clinic.

22. Program Management and Parent counselling Training

Every program manager, coordinator and counsellor undergoes a week long training program to be equipped to lead and succeed in the clubfoot disability eradication program. Counsellors, who also serve as program coordinators have multiple responsibilities including counselling parents, documenting the treatment progress, building partnership, raiseing awareness and mobilizing resources. Like a woman could be a daughter, a mother and a wife at the same time, likewise in the clubfoot management, the same person has a multi-tasking responsibility. Counsellors work on three major responsibilities like clinic management, program management and resource mobilization.

The program management and the parent counselling cannot be separated. The person involved in the clinic management has to have the ability to work with the doctors who are professionals and experts as well as the parents majority of whom have had very little education. Parents in public hospitals are generally extremely poor whose priority in life includes meeting the needs of the household every day. The counsellor has to understand the treatment progress by working closely with the doctors and disseminate the required information to the parents through parent teaching printed materials that includes visuals. It is important to keep the interest level of parents high to comply with the protocol of the Ponseti treatment. The training program helps them understand their role and s them to be successful in working with doctors and the parents.

The counsellors like any general public come with less or no knowledge about clubfoot. It is important that the counsellors understand basic information about spectrum of clubfoot, Ponseti method, weekly manipulation and casting, tenotomy, Pirani score and the importance of long term bracing. All these topics are taught to the counsellors so that they serve in each clinic as Ponseti's protocol officer. The counsellors help the parents to complete the treatment as per the Ponseti technique. It is the responsibility of the counsellors to make sure that each child enrolled for clubfoot treatment completes the treatment and follow-up for five years successfully. The program coordinators and counsellors have a mandate to ensure compulsory and complete treatment for children born with clubfoot in the geographical area of service. It is also their responsibility to ensure all relevant information is uploaded in the electronic registry.

Each clinic location has at least one counsellor and it is this counsellor who has to focus on maintaining minimum stock of brace, and other materials based on the checklist. Counsellors are also trained to monitor the performance of the clinic to match the minimum required quality in care. Since the clubfoot clinics functions only once a week, the counsellor finds time to raise awareness in local school, colleges, 'aganwadis' etc. Counsellors are also trained to carry out regular home visits to help parents comply with the protocol of the Ponseti method. Ultimately the counsellor's role is to make sure that each child enrolled for treatment gets quality care and each and every one of them completes five years of follow-up with foot abduction brace.

23. Partnership with State and National Governments

Ownership and support of the local government is vital for the success of large clubfoot management programs at the state, province, union territory or national level. CURE India's policy is to work only with public/ government hospitals and medical colleges managed by the State or Central government because the poorest of the poor visit the public hospitals for any treatment or medical care and the priority of CURE initiative is to serve the poor who cannot afford paid treatment. Healthcare provided at the public hospitals is free of cost to people below the poverty line. CURE also provides what is missing in the public healthcare systems and hospitals (refresher training to doctors on the Ponseti method, counsellors to follow-up, brace, documentation and helpline support). Designated weekly clubfoot clinics are established with the approval and guidance of each of the State governments. A memorandum of understanding is signed with each of the 27 out of 29 states in India, where the doctors are trained and designated clinics are established. Trained counsellors are appointed to counsel and teach the parents who bring children for clubfoot treatment. Counsellors also help doctors maintain medical records electronically and braces are distributed free of cost to each child by the counsellors.

In the partnership with State governments the role of CURE is to

i. Provide annual refresher training to healthcare professionals who participate in the treatment of clubfoot.

ii. Maintain medical records (electronically and manually) for every child enrolled in the program.

iii. Appoint counsellors to teach parents the protocol on Ponseti method, maintain medical records, distribute braces and attend 24X7 clubfoot helpline.

iv. Distribute foot abduction brace for every child free of cost.

v. Manage programs by appointing program managers and coordinators to work in coordination with the respective state government.

vi.   Establish and maintain 24x7 state level clubfoot helpline.

In the public- private partnership, the role of the state government is to

i.   Depute dedicated doctors for every clinic who attend the refresher training and provide quality Ponseti care to the children.

ii.   Ensure availability of quality treatment materials like plaster of Paris (PoP), soft ban, cotton and the materials required for tenotomy procedure.

iii.   Provide clinic space where counsellors meet the parents, store brace & medical records, doctors consult the children, provide casting etc.

iv.   Use the existing community health awareness and screening team to identify and refer children born with clubfoot for free treatment from the designated clubfoot clinics in the state.

There are ten points that are required to establish ideal clubfoot clinics and ensure successful completion of treatment. In the program in India, four of the components come from government side (designated doctor, clinic/counselling/office space, treatment materials and using the health volunteers and other works in RBSK identify and refer children to the weekly clubfoot clinic) and six of them (regular refresher training on Ponseti method, maintaining medical records, providing counsellors, distribution of foot abduction brace, 24x7 Helpline, program management) come from CURE. Ten points put together make a successful clubfoot program.

In the partnership with the central government CURE works very closely with the National Health Mission (NHM). The Rashtriya Bal Swasthya Karyakram (RBSK) the National Child Health Program of NHM has included clubfoot as one of the birth defects to be identified and treated compulsorily. In several states, when children are identified for treatment for clubfoot, the information is shared with CURE and the counsellors follow-up with the parents to ensure successful treatment from the designated clubfoot clinic. The shared vision in this public-private partnership program is to see India free from the disability of clubfoot.

24. Rotary's leadership in Clubfoot disability eradication

In India the fight to eradicate polio was successfully carried out by a powerful partnership that emerged between Rotary and the Indian Government both at the State and the National level. Now that the fight against polio has been won, Rotary club is spearheading the battle against clubfoot disability. The goal is to get as many children as possible to the treatment facilities for free treatment. Rotary clubs in Bangalore and Delhi are actively leading the Clubfoot India program.

Rtn S. A. Chandran of Essay Foundation, Rtn Praful Kumar, Rtn Krishnamurthy, Rtn Suresh Mahanandi and Rtn Chourappa from Bangalore Rotary District continue to be the driving force to include the clubfoot program in the agenda of Rotary clubs in South India. Prof. Dr Iris Devadason, a retired English teacher, dedicated her retired life to create paintings to be sold to raise funds and awareness to support the cause of clubfoot. An exhibition of her paintings was held in Bangalore in Dec. 2010 that inspired the Rotary members to include clubfoot in their service agenda. Apart from financial support, the rotary volunteers regularly visit weekly clubfoot clinic to encourage the parents to complete the treatment.

Rotary clubs in Delhi have adopted designated clubfoot clinics. The model of Rotary adopting clinics emerged out of the active leadership of Rtn Amarnath Goyal, who for the last four years has completely dedicated his life for children born with clubfoot. Rtn Amarnath Goyal was inspired to serve children born with clubfoot after meeting Dr Mathew Varghese in his busy clubfoot clinic in June 2012. Rtn Amarnath successfully encouraged Rotary Clubfoot of Delhi South (RCDS) to consider clubfoot as a priority project of the club. CURE and RCDS signed an MoU in Nov 2012 during the Diwali celebration of the club members. The 'celebration of light' of the club spread rays of hope to thousands of children and in four years, five Rotary clubs in and around Delhi have adopted five designated clubfoot clinics. These designated clubfoot clinics have Rotary members volunteering every week at the clinic, interacting with the parents, encouraging doctors, and inspiring children with gifts, snacks and sweets. The foot abduction braces in these clinics are financially sponsored by Rotary clubs.

A MoU has also been signed between CURE and Rotary in Lucknow in June 2016 and Rotary Club of Delhi Midtown in Aug 2016. Rtn Sanjay Khanna, Rtn Vinod Bansal, Rtn Dr Subramanian, Rtn Pradeep Bahri, Rtn Rishab Jain, Rtn Pradeep Kumar, Rtn Pradeep Gupta continue to spearhead the Rotary clubfoot disability eradication program. Rotary clubs in Tamil Nadu supported clubfoot program through Rtn Vennimalai and Rtn Mythly Muralidharan.

The role of Rotary in the eradication of disability from clubfoot comprises raising of public awareness on the prevalence of clubfoot and the availability of free treatment and raising funds to support foot abduction brace and ensuring treatment for all children identified with clubfoot. A campaign with the motto "Treat Clubfoot Today" was launched in February 2013 during the First National Clubfoot Conference at New Delhi that was inaugurated by the Hon. Vice President of India Shri. Hameed Ansari in the presence of Delhi Chief Minister Smt. Sheila Dikshit. The active participation of Rotary members in the clubfoot management program is a sign of success in our aim to eradicate disability from clubfoot globally.

Inner wheel actively supports clubfoot program in the National Capital region of Delhi. Midtown Inner wheel club is financially sponsoring several children in their treatment. Mrs Namrata Wadhwana initiated this partnership along with a team of active leaders like Ms Neelu Khanna, Ms Abha Gupta, Ms Shashi Kumar, Ms Kamla Aggarwal, Ms Santosh Bindal and Ms Meena Jain.

25. Conclusion: Many missions but only one Vision

The only vision in the clubfoot management program is to see this world free of disability from clubfoot. The immediate goal is to ensure compulsory and complete treatment for clubfoot across the globe. If every child born with clubfoot gets treatment and every child getting into the treatment completes it successfully, our dream will come true: the dream to make clubfoot deformity history. Success depends on how effectively the healthcare professionals, voluntary organisations, government systems and parents come together determined with the same vision and goal.

The ever-growing myths and misunderstanding around clubfoot and its treatment will diminish faster the closer we move towards our goal. Let the wisdom gained so far on clubfoot management and the progress we could achieve enable more children to benefit from the advantage of the conservative Ponseti technique.

My sincere wish is that a day will soon come when the cause for clubfoot is known and the birth deformity is prevented for ever. Until then it is my prayer that this book may help many children across the globe get compulsory and complete treatment for clubfoot so that not even one child is left without treatment.

V. Frequently Asked Questions (FAQ)

There are many questions mothers, grandmothers and other relatives ask when they bring their child for treatment. This session is intended to provide answers for all those frequently asked questions (FAQ).

i. What causes clubfoot? Why is my child born with clubfoot?

The reason for clubfoot is unknown. Since the cause is unknown, one cannot say that mother or father or anyone else in the family is the reason for a child to be born with clubfoot. Mothers should not feel guilty for giving birth to a child with clubfoot. There are many theories regarding what causes clubfoot but nothing has been verified so far to be the one specific reason for children to be born with clubfoot.

ii. When is the right time to start treatment for clubfoot?

For at least two reasons the treatment should start immediately after the birth. One, the foot is tender when the child is small and the treatment of manipulation and casting becomes easy. So the treatment should start if not immediately after the birth, at least any time before two to three months, so that the foot is corrected and the child is ready to walk at the walking stage. The second reason for early treatment is to prevent any social stigma attached to the family and the child. Because of the growing misunderstanding about clubfoot, children are given nicknames and parents and family are excluded from community activities and festivals. To prevent this social stigma, it is important that children get the feet corrected as early as possible.

iii. What is the best treatment for clubfoot?

The best treatment available at present globally is the non-surgical method called the Ponseti method. This Ponseti method is a conservative method where the foot is corrected with weekly plaster casting. The final cast is applied after a minor procedure called tenotomy. The weekly plaster casting is applied for four to six weeks depending on the severity of the clubfoot and the age of the child. After tenotomy which is the cutting of a tendon, the cast remains for three weeks. Once the foot is completely corrected, foot abduction brace (special shoe with abduction bar) is provided to prevent relapse. The child has to wear this brace 23 hours a day first for three months and subsequently night and nap time bracing for four-five years.

iv. Why is Ponseti method better than surgical correction?

In the Ponseti method, the foot is corrected with manipulation, casting and tenotomy and the corrected foot is maintained in that position with long term bracing to prevent recurrence, whereas in the surgical method the bones and tissues are damaged to attain the correction. The bones even after breaking grow normally whereas the tissues do not grow in the same speed as bones. Thus the surgically corrected foot results in a stiff foot which is not flexible. Once the foot is inflexible, children cannot wear normal shoes. Studies show that the children who have undergone Ponseti method do not have pain or any complications, whereas the children who have undergone surgery always suffer pain and stiffness in the ankle and foot. There are instances where the foot is amputated after severe pain and complication as a result of multiple surgeries.

v. Ponseti method is known as non-surgical method; then why tenotomy?

Tenotomy is not surgery: it is a minor procedure where the tendon is cut. Only local anaesthetic is given to the child and there are no stitches given after this procedure. The tendon that is cut regenerates naturally in three weeks. So this procedure cannot be equated to any surgery and that is why the Ponseti method is called a non-surgical method. Compared to the popular surgical method, where children have to undergo major surgery to correct the deformed foot the Ponseti method is truly a non-surgical method.

vii. What if in a bilateral clubfoot one foot is ready for tenotomy and the other is not corrected?

Both the feet continue to get weekly casting. Casting in one foot is to maintain the correction whereas casting in the other foot is to get more correction so that both the feet can go for tenotomy together. After the tenotomy the cast remains for three weeks and then the brace is applied to maintain the correction.

vii. Is clubfoot hereditary?

There are 15% chances for parents with clubfoot to have children born with clubfoot. So, if there are 100 parents only around 15 parents will have children born with clubfoot.

viii. Why does my child require a special shoe?

Clubfoot is a birth deformity and there are chances that the corrected foot goes back to the original deformed position. After correcting the clubfoot with Ponseti method, to prevent the foot from going back to a disabled position, foot abduction braces are used. A special shoe is given not because there is any disability in the child, but to prevent any recurrence after the conservative treatment.

ix. When the foot looks corrected and normal why follow-up for five years?

Corrected clubfoot looks normal but it is like a dog's tail. When we hold it straight it remains strait but when we release it , it goes to the original position. In four to six weeks correction is achieved in a foot that was twisted inward and upward. To maintain the correction it is important that the foot is kept in the corrected position with foot abduction brace for four to five years (first three months 23 hours a day and then night and nap time for four to five years).

Earlier the protocol for follow up with the brace was for two to three years. Later the scholars and researchers involved with Ponseti method learnt that children who were left without foot abduction braces after three years suffered a relapse. The follow up time was increased to four years and at present the international standard for follow up using foot abduction brace for clubfoot is five years.

x. Why special shoes to be worn night and nap time?

The human bone grows during the night and so it is important that the bones grow in the corrected position. So night time bracing is scientifically compulsory in the treatment for clubfoot. Nevertheless naptime bracing is also made compulsory for practical reasons. Any child will cry when a brace is applied and they miss sleep time during night. When they miss sleep at night, children sleep longer time during the day. When this process of less sleep during night and long sleep during day happens for several days and weeks, the children end up sleeping very few hours or no sleep during night and long hours of sleep during day. This could cause relapse because the corrected foot is let free for more hours during night. To prevent this crisis, parents are taught to help their children wear the brace during night and nap time. In this process the children associate sleep with bracing and they overcome the initial irritation to wear foot abduction brace.

xi. Why the foot is kept in 70 degree external rotation or abduction?

The foot is like a boat. It has three movements that happen simultaneously. Yawing, pitching and rolling all three movements happen at the same time in boats. The foot also yaws, pitches and rolls. So it is not enough to get the foot that was inward and upward straight but a 70 degree external rotation is required and this is achieved during the casting and tenotomy to ensure all three movements.

xii. How much does it cost to completely correct clubfoot?

In public hospitals where CURE is partnering the treatment is completely free. The casting materials are available free of cost in government hospitals and the trained doctors are available who provide free consultation and treatment. In addition CURE complements the work by providing parent counselling, documentation and free distribution of foot abduction brace.

xiii. How expensive is the treatment for clubfoot in a private hospital?

If the child is given Ponseti method of treatment, for casting the charges range from Rs 100 to Rs 5000 depending on the hospital and location. For tenotomy the cost ranges from Rs 500 to Rs 20,000. However, if the child undergoes surgery for the correction of clubfoot, the cost ranges from 20,000 to 3,00,000/- (information from parents)

xiv. Why does CURE work only with government hospitals?

Affordable and accessible healthcare is a constitutional right and the public hospitals in India provide healthcare free of cost. The poorest of the poor visit the public hospitals for any treatment and medical care and the priority of CURE initiative is to serve the poor who cannot afford paid treatment. For any deformity or disability to be eradicated, the active leadership of the government is mandatory. The role of CURE as a voluntary organisation is to serve as a private partner in the Public – Private Partnership Program.

xv. How are the records maintained for children enrolled for treatment?

Medical records are maintained manually and electronically. Detailed folders with space to mark the Pirani score is used in the entire designated weekly clubfoot clinic. The electronic record that is maintained is called International Clubfoot Registry.

xvi. What is the basic information the general public should know about clubfoot?

Every individual should know the prevalence of clubfoot and the treatment available for the correction of clubfoot. Differences between clubfoot and polio, the Ponseti method of clubfoot correction and importance of long-term bracing are some of the topics the general public should know.